Dr C. Norman Shealy MD, PhD, is founder of the Shealy Institute in Springfield, Missouri, a centre for comprehensive health care and pain and stress management. He is founder of The American Holistic Medical Association. His previous books include *The Pain Game*, *The Creation of Health* and *Miracles Do Happen*, and he was consultant editor on *The Complete Family Guide to Alternative Medicine*, *The Complete Family Guide to Natural Home Remedies* and *The Illustrated Encyclopaedia of Healing Remedies*. This book is written with the help of a grant from the Charlson Research Foundation.

C. Norman Shealy MD PhD

90 days

TO STRESS-FREE LIVING

a day-by-day health plan including
exercises, diet and relaxation techniques

ISBN 1-84333-384-8

A catalogue record for this book is available from
the British Library

First published in 2002 by
Vega
64 Brewery Road
London, N7 9NT

A member of **Chrysalis** Books plc

Visit our website at www.chrysalisbooks.co.uk

Printed in Great Britain by
Creative Print and Design (Wales)

Front cover main and central images
and back cover image © Digital Vision Ltd.

Contents

Introduction:
An Overview of Stress

The quality of every aspect of our lives is affected by the state of our health. So perhaps the first thing we should do is take some time to consider some of the factors which influence our health.

Health is a wonderfully complex interaction between genes and environment, between attitude and behaviour, between lifestyle and chance. About 98 per cent of infants born to healthy parents are healthy. Health is the *natural*, normal state of being; most often we remain healthy unless we lead a stressful life. As we progress into adulthood, it is increasingly important that we create a healthy lifestyle.

Experts agree that *at least* 85 per cent of all illnesses are the result of lifestyle. Thus, most illness is avoidable. On the other hand, developing and maintaining a healthy lifestyle requires active commitment to living certain ideas. *90 Days to Stress-free Living* provides a framework within which to begin living that life.

After this brief overview of the principles of health, we offer you a daily programme which will establish a habit of *living* health. Ninety days is chosen because three months is a minimal time in which to develop a habit.

Stress

The Canadian physician, Dr Hans Selye, identified stress as a major cause of disease. Selye's earliest work primarily involved physical and chemical stressors, although he later looked at emotional stress as well. We now know that electromagnetic energy is also stressful, as is nuclear radiation.

1

Selye stated that any of these stressors causes an alarm reaction, making the body respond as if a major life-threatening crisis had occurred. This was perhaps most useful back in the days when we had to avoid tigers and other such 'natural' threats. Selye emphasized that the first time we are exposed to a stressor, we may have a reaction in which adrenaline output doubles, but this usually returns to normal when we respond to the threat by either fighting or running away. Under normal circumstances, a balancing mechanism occurs which restores us to our baseline level of adrenaline output. When the stressor is nicotine, such as from a cigarette, the return to normal occurs ordinarily within 10 to 15 minutes. When it is caffeine from a cup of coffee, it may take a minimum of 4 hours, and up to 30 hours to return to baseline.

If the body receives the same stressor on a regular basis, it no longer responds with a marked outpouring of adrenaline. This is considered adaptation, but Selye pointed out that every time we adapt to a stressor, we lower our tolerance to new stress, and at some point our ability to adapt becomes compromised. This leads to maladaptation, at which point we develop major stress symptoms, and eventually physical exhaustion and illness.

Selye also emphasized the cumulative effects of minute amounts of stress. For instance, one cigarettte doubles our adrenaline output, but a third of a cigarette does not cause much change. However, a third of a cigarette, a third of a cup of coffee and a doughnut would trigger an alarm reaction.

Significant known stressors are:

Physical	Chemical
Allergens	Alcohol
Inactivity	Caffeine
Inadequate light	Infection
Temperature extremes	Nicotine
Toxins	Nutrition imbalance
Trauma	Sugar

Emotional
Anger
Anxiety
Depression
Fear
Guilt
Inadequate sleep
Pain

Electromagnetic
Airplanes
Automobiles
Computer printers
Computers
Fluorescent lights
Refrigerators
Television

Nuclear radiation
Major effects upon:
   DNA/gene
   Immune function
   Thyroid function

Spiritual
Concerns about:
   Ethics
   Existence
   Morals
   Purpose

The body's natural coping mechanism for stress is primarily physical (fight or flight), but with many of the stressors listed above, it is obvious that we do not respond with the balancing mechanism of physical activity. It has been known now for some 70 years that deep relaxation is also a significant antidote to stress. So as well as avoiding stressors, 15 to 20 minutes of deep relaxation twice a day can lower the entire 24-hour production of adrenaline by 50 per cent. It is also known that the higher the number of stress symptoms, the greater the chance of having a disease. An increase of more than five or six stress symptoms is evidence of increasing maladaptation. Check against the following list of symptoms to see how well you are coping with stress!

SYMPTOM INDEX

– Anxiety or worry
– Back or shoulder pain
– Being extremely shy
– Biting your nails
– Breathing problems
– Change in sense of taste
– Coated tongue

– Cold hands or feet
– Constipation
– Coughing spells
– Dental problems
– Depressed mood
– Diarrhoea
– Difficulty in concentrating

3

- Difficulty in swallowing
- Digestive problems
- Dizziness
- Enlarged tonsils
- Epilepsy
- Excess belching
- Excess hunger
- Fatigue, low energy
- Feel lonely or sad
- Feeling bloated
- Feelings of worthlessness or guilt
- Frequent colds
- Frequent crying
- Frequent stomach trouble
- Frequent urination at night
- Getting angry easily
- Headaches
- Hearing problems
- Heartburn
- Heart problems
- Haemorrhoids
- Hernia or rupture
- High or low blood pressure
- Indecisiveness
- Insomnia
- Intestinal worms
- Itching or burning skin
- Kidney or bladder disease
- Leg cramps
- Loss of appetite
- Lumps or swelling in neck
- Motion sickness
- Nausea
- Nervous exhaustion
- Other bowel problems
- Oversleeping
- Overweight or underweight
- Painful feet
- Peptic ulcer
- Recurrent thoughts of death or suicide
- Sedentary
- Sexual problems
- Shortness of breath
- Significant weight loss or gain
- Sore or sensitive tongue
- Sore throat or hoarseness
- Stiff or painful muscles or joints
- Stuttering or stammering
- Surgery within the past year
- Swelling in armpits or groin
- Teeth or gum problems
- Tendency to be too hot or too cold
- Tendency to shake or tremble
- Urinary problems
- Varicose veins
- Vision problems
- Yellow jaundice

For women only:

- Difficult or heavy menses
- Having had a hysterectomy
- Hot flushes
- Lumpy breasts
- Taking birth control pills

(in the last year)
- Having hormone replacement therapy
- PMS
- Vaginal discharge

Other factors which markedly increase your stress levels are being indoors in 'managed' air, not getting a minimum of one hour of natural daylight per day, and a general discontent with life. This discontent includes what I call any 'unfinished business' – anything which causes clear-cut fear, anger, guilt, anxiety or depression.

Genetics

Once you've chosen your parents you cannot significantly improve your genetic factors. And there are thousands of them. Indeed, a majority of illnesses have some genetic predilection, although it is often small. For instance, epilepsy occurs in about 1 per cent of people; but, in the family of an epileptic, the incidence is 3 per cent of family members. Hypertension, asthma, diabetes, rheumatoid arthritis, heart disease, and many forms of cancer have varying genetic influences. Virtually all illnesses, however, are much more strongly influenced by smoking, alcohol, obesity, poor nutrition, and inadequate physical exercise than they are by genetics.

In reality, *attitude* is the single most critical health determinant; for attitude determines one's habits – even to the choice of reading this book and making a commitment to health.

Attitude

In her inspirational book *The Spiritual Life*, Evelyn Underhill, a Christian mystic, says that living the spiritual life is not living in a monastery or nunnery; it is 'the attitude you hold in your mind when you're down on your knees cleaning the steps'. And indeed it is the attitude you hold when you are down on your knees cleaning the toilet, or when you're dealing with the most obnoxious, irritating aspects of life.

Attitude is probably influenced more by your *perception* of your infancy and early childhood than by all other subsequent events. In reality, there are only two extremes of attitude – positive or negative. A positive attitude reflects good self-esteem or the 'I'm OK' concept of Tom Harris, author of *I'm OK, You're OK*. A negative attitude is more like the 'Bah, humbug' of Scrooge, disparaging even the most sacred of events.

A negative attitude results from a *perception* of either abandonment or abuse – a feeling that one is unlovable, bad or evil. In Western society, in fact, one's entry into the world is likely to include abandonment *and* abuse: you're slapped on the back and taken away from your mother! Undoubtedly that initial shock is reinforced by multiple events in early life, many of which the adult may not *intend* as hurtful or harmful. The arrival of other children, or perceived favouritism of one child over another or the parents' irritation with life's stresses all may contribute to *feelings* of being inadequate or undeserving.

Threats or negative comments by adults may combine to create a basic negative attitude or *fear*. In assessing *your* fears, be aware that there are only *five* possible fears:

death
illness (invalidism/pain)
poverty (insecurity)
abandonment (loss of love)
meaning (purpose/moral values/sense of justice).

The usual normal response to fear is survival which by instinct should lead to either fight (anger) or flight (divorce); unfortunately, fear may also lead to 'freeze' (depression, guilt). Anxiety is likely to accompany all these reactions. Actually, anxiety is really a synonym for fear itself.

Thus there are only four negative *feelings* as the result of an attitude of fear:

anxiety
anger
guilt
depression.

All other negative feelings are actually *synonyms* of these four.

And always keep in mind that fear is always the result of a *perception* of either abuse or abandonment.

In reality, we have very few *needs*, namely: air, water, food, clothes, shelter, and nurturing. If adequately supplied with these essentials throughout childhood, in adolescence one will develop additional needs for sexual experience and freedom. If properly nurtured early, these needs will be much more easily met in a healthy way.

When nurturing has been inadequate for the provision of secure self-esteem, anxiety develops. When nurturing has been negative (abusive), anger is a natural result. When nurturing has been extremely lacking, depression is likely. And when nurturing has been petulant or accusative, guilt is the result.

As individuals mature, if nurturing has been inadequate, and self-esteem is low, then neurotic symptoms increase and self-esteem substitutes may be craved: sex, money, power. Attempts to gain these self-esteem substitutes may lead to profligate sexuality, great fear of poverty, and various cravings which can manifest as greed, obsession, or even stealing. Attempts to use power as a substitute for self-worth can range from accepting an abused co-dependent relationship to the most aggressive misuse of power in forms of intimidation, and serious corruption, or brutality.

Ultimately, as adults, we must recognize that we are responsible for our attitude and our behaviour. Once basic needs are met, the mature adult derives more pleasure from *giving* nurturing than from all other needs. Desires for excessive sex, money, and power are replaced by desires to do good to self and others – unconditional love. Thus one major goal for self-healing is to reach a state where the dominant attitude is positive, joyous, and loving.

From this perspective, at some juncture, one begins to perceive that most pain is a failure to accept things as they are or a refusal to accept reality. This maturing insight does not require one to accept abuse; quite the contrary. As one works towards the transcendent

7

will, or the will of the soul, it becomes obvious that there are only three possible solutions to fear and all the feelings it engenders. These solutions are fight (assertion), flight (divorce), or forgiveness/acceptance (going for sainthood).

When you are threatened, you have a right to be angry and to fight back. Your assertion may be through conversation, argument, lawsuits, or physical battle.

In some situations, fighting is inappropriate or unsuccessful. If abuse continues or is intolerable, then you have a responsibility to flee – divorce the intolerable with joy. Rejoice, as you leave, that you do not have to put up with abuse.

When the situation is not correctable or divorceable, then your only option is acceptance and forgiveness, while moving towards positive goals. Any continuing anger, anxiety, guilt, or depression is only a self-induced, energy-depleting stress.

When you resolve all your fear, you are left detached and non-judgmental, with no need to know why. You are at peace.

The purpose of *90 Days to Stress-free Living* is to assist you in reaching this transcendent goal. Each day for three months you will have an opportunity to concentrate upon physical, emotional, and attitudinal harmony.

The Golden Rule

There is only one great law of life: treat others well or they will get even with you!

Love yourself – and love others. Desire to do good to everyone. It is not easy, but it is soul satisfying.

Before you begin the daily programme, it is essential that you recognize also that physical exercise is one of the greatest known stress reducers. Adequate physcial exercise increases your *tolerance* for social, emotional, and even chemical stress.

It is also important to recognize that nutrition is a key element in health. The essentials of good nutrition will be outlined after those for physical exercise.

Physical Exercise

Physical stressors are mostly inactivity and accidents. Barometric pressure changes and electromagnetic pollution undoubtedly contribute to our stress levels, but are not so measurable. Actually, adequate physical exercise is the single greatest stress reducer known.

Adequate (optimal) physical exercise means getting 45 to 60 aerobics points per week. (I'll tell you how to do it later.) Ideally, optimal health requires a minimum of four and a maximum of six days of exercise per week. Thus I encourage you to plan for 10 to 15 aerobics points each exercise period. Of course, you will take at least three months to reach this exercise intensity and, if in poor shape initially, you may take six months.

Which of the following are you willing to develop?

Walking

4 miles in 60 min. = 11 points
5 miles in 75 min. = 14 points

Jogging

3 miles in 36 min. = 11 points
4 miles in 48 min. = 15 points
3 miles in 30 min. = 14 points

Jogging on a trampoline

120 steps/min. = 1 point/4 min.
180 steps/min. = 1 point/3 min.
240 steps/min. = 1 point/2 min.

Stationary Bike

At 35 mph = 1 point/3 min.

Racquetball

10 points/60 min.

If you prefer swimming or some other sport, check one of Dr Kenneth Cooper's many books on aerobic exercise.

In addition to cardiovascular physical exercise you need *limbering*. I strongly recommend the following limbering exercises. Remember that these should be comfortable and fun. Start with what you can do easily and build gradually. Practise the limbering exercises every day. By the time you can do 21 repetitions, these exercises should take you no more than 10 minutes.

Twirling

With the arms stretched out at shoulder height, turn clockwise (towards the right). Start by doing not more than 2 or 3 twirls and build up gradually over a period of 2 or 3 weeks to 21 twirls a day.

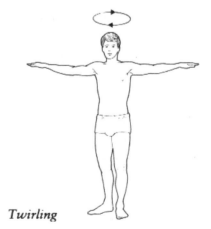

Twirling

Head and Leg Raises

Lying flat on your back on a firm surface with your hands beside your buttocks, take a deep breath in and, as you breathe out, raise your legs straight up into the air. At the same time raise your head up as if you were going to touch your head to your knees. Knees are kept straight. Then, as legs and head are lowered to the floor, take another deep breath. Again, start off with 2 or 3 exercises and build up over a period of 2 or 3 weeks to a total of 21.

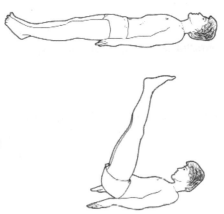

Head and leg raise

Back Arches

On a carpeted floor, keep your body erect while kneeling. Bend your head forward on the chest and take a deep breath. As you breathe out, bend your head back as far as it will go, keeping your thighs straight up, arching your head and back maximally. You may put your hands behind the lower part of your buttocks to give additional stability. Start with 2 or 3 repetitions and build to 21.

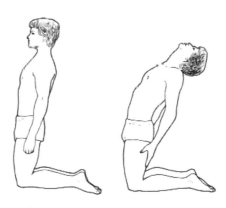

Back arches

11

The Table

While sitting with your legs straight out in front, put your palms flat on the floor directly beside your buttocks. Bend your head forward as you breathe out, raise your knees up into the air to make your thighs parallel with the floor and your calves perpendicular to the floor. At the same time, arch your head and neck backwards and breathe out. This makes your body, from the shoulders down to the knees, parallel with the floor and gives the appearance of your body being a table. Start with 2 repetitions and build to 21.

The table

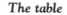
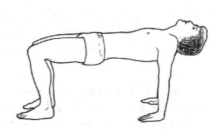
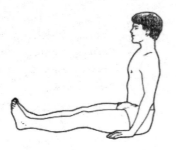

Modified Cobra

Put yourself in position as if you were doing push-ups, with your toes supporting your body at one end and your palms flat down on the

Modified cobra

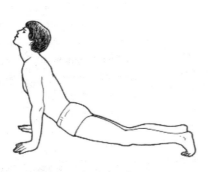
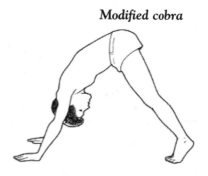

floor at the other end. Extend your head back as far as it will go, arching your upper back, keeping your knees straight. Take a deep breath. As you breathe out, bend your head forward and bring your buttocks straight up into the air, keeping your knees straight. Start with 2 repetitions and build to 21.

Sit-ups

In addition, sit-ups with your knees bent are excellent for abdominal strengthening, very important in preventing back injuries.

If you walk, jog or use a trampoline, add weights or a dumb-bell as these can add great extra exercise to your upper body and heart. You can start with 1 pound (0.5 kg) in each hand and build up to 10 (5 kg). Even simple dumb-bells can be used.

Nutrition

Good nutrition is simple but not easy. Many people are addicted to fast, fat, and sweet. None of these is necessary. *Optimal* nutrition means you eat a wide variety of *real* food, avoiding highly processed foods such as those containing or described as:

processed	sugar
hardened	corn sweetener/syrup
hydrogenated	bleached
partially	'enriched' (is very deficient)
substitute	flavoured.
artificially	

Breakfast Ideas

1. Low or non-fat yogurt with a bit of honey, fresh fruit, and a handful of toasted almonds or cashews.

2. Wholegrain bread with natural peanut butter (sugar free, low salt) plus juice or fruit, or with cheese.
3. Oatmeal or other wholegrain cereal with an egg or cheese or nuts.
4. Eggs and toast. Unless you have familial hypercholesteraemia, eggs are good for you – in moderation. Certainly I can find no scientific evidence that 7 eggs a week harm anyone. Indeed, for most people, 14 per week is okay. Check your cholesterol before making that decision.

Lunch and Supper

Soups
Salads
Veggies galore
Fruits, nuts, seeds
4oz (100 g) of lean fish, chicken, turkey, or red meat (but avoid beef more than twice a week)
Wholegrain breads, rice, potatoes.

If you crave pizza, try a wholewheat base with lots of veggie toppings and enjoy it – but not more than twice a week.

In general, avoid most fast food restaurants.

Habits

Nutrition, exercise, and attitudes – these are the basic habits. All require willpower. As William Lee Wilbanks has emphasized in his great article, 'The New Obscenity', the only solution to any undesirable habit is development of willpower. You can help yourself if you will. Smoking, alcohol, drugs, obesity, laziness, inactivity, poor nutrition, and even depression, all can be overcome through active practice of willpower. Our three-month programme will centre on development of will.

Sex

As did Wilhelm Reich, I believe sexual orgasm is a natural, normal, and essential aspect of health. Reich was a contemporary of Freud and is considered by many to have been one of the most influential psychiatrists of all time. And I agree with Reich that one must learn to please oneself first in order to know one's sensual capabilities. I strongly recommend that you read and heed the excellent advice/practice of these books: *Masturbation, Tantra and Self Love* by Margo Woods (for everyone); *Male Sexuality* by Bernie Zilbergeld (for men); *Our Bodies, Ourselves* by the Boston Women's Health Book Collection (for women).

I do not recommend promiscuity. If you have a truly loved one, then sex can be more fulfilling. If you do not, it can be fun and healthy – with yourself! I believe sex is a spiritual connection. As such, it is a sacred part of life.

Relaxation

The thrust of this self-healing programme is stress reduction at an attitudinal, physical, and chemical level. In addition to avoiding chemical stress and using physical exercise to improve stress, there is another great stress antidote known and studied throughout this century. As early as 1925, Edmund Jacobson, in his classic book *Progressive Relaxation*, demonstrated that 80 per cent of all 'psychosomatic illnesses' could be controlled by regular deep relaxation. He demonstrated, in thousands of individuals, the homeostatic (balancing) effects of 30 minutes of deep relaxation. Blood pressure, pulse, and all stress reactions are moderated by consistent daily practice of deep relaxation.

In the 1970s Benson led modern scientific investigation of the beneficial effects of relaxation. His work was largely summarized in his best-selling book, *The Relaxation Response*. The most critical foundation for relaxation is the focus of attention or mental concentration upon any thought that is non-stressful. Thus, focus on a word such as 'one' or 'love'. Indeed, *any* word said repetitively can lead to relaxation. Most music can be relaxing, as can watching nature, a candle, a repetitive light, observing breathing, or listening to a repetitive sound. All relaxation, no matter how it is achieved, leads to:

- decreased blood pressure
- slower, more regular heart rate
- decreased electrical frequency of the brain ('alpha' rhythm)
- decreased muscle tension
- decreased insulin requirement
- decreased 'adrenalin' production.

In fact, deep relaxation done 20 minutes twice a day leads to a 50 per cent reduction in total insulin requirement and in total adrenalin production for the entire 24 hour period. And most relaxation techniques also lead to increased levels of beta endorphin, the natural narcotic or feel-good chemical.

The combination of physical exercise, relaxation, and working on achieving the right attitude offers a total health programme which cannot be achieved without personal effort. But that effort will pay off handsomely with improved health and well-being. Fortunately, the entire programme should be fun and feel good.

Retraining the Nervous System

The most important concept to know, understand, and absorb is that all influences have physical results, although your body may be influenced physically, chemically, or emotionally.

Physical influences include such simple factors as the pressure of glasses over your eyes, a watch on your wrist, a ring on your finger, clothes on your body, the pressure of your body down upon your buttocks in sitting, upon your feet in standing, and so on. It also includes touching outside objects; but when other people touch you, then it becomes both a physical and an emotional feeling.

A wide variety of chemicals influence your feelings as well. For instance, alcohol, coffee, sugar, sugary drinks, and many drugs will alter the physiology (the chemistry and electricity) of your body so that you may become more or less sensitive to feelings.

Finally, there are emotional feelings. And emotional feelings are the physical reactions in your body to joy or fear.

Ultimately, what you perceive as feelings are either feelings that individual parts of the body are OK, that is, they feel good, or feelings of discomfort. The feelings of discomfort range from tension or tightness all the way to the most intense of these, which is pain. At times, when a great deal of stress has been focused upon one part of the body, you 'lose' feelings there, even without nerve damage. This is caused by a psychological or/and electrical blockage which stops information flowing to and from that part of the body, as well as causing decreased blood flow.

The first step, then, is to learn actually to *feel* the body properly. This means tuning in to your body and just getting the sensory feedback or awareness from your body. Then, you need to learn to alter or change feelings, and in this way gain control over them. The techniques for changing body feelings are:

1. Talking to the body. For instance, 'My hand is warm'. If you do this long enough, your hand will warm up.
2. Image changes. For instance, imagining the sun beaming down upon your hand will assist the process of warming it.
3. Feel the pulsations of your heartbeat in that area. Actually, this happens almost automatically if you're not tense in a body area. Do not ever allow yourself to feel the pulsations inside your head, however, as that could cause a vascular or migraine type headache. But in every other part of the body pulsing is associated with the state of relaxation.
4. Tense a part of the body; for instance, make a fist. Compare the feelings of tension with those of relaxation as you relax and let go. The simple process of physically contracting and then relaxing a part of the body changes feelings.

17

5. Focus a feeling of love upon the body. This allows that part of the body to feel nurtured and OK.
6. Breathing. Collect and release. If you feel a part of your body that is tense, imagine collecting that tension as you breathe in and releasing it as you breathe out. This can markedly reduce the amount of tension in that part of your body.
7. Breathing through the skin. Pretending that you are breathing through the surface of the skin will change the feelings in that part of your body. Doing this for 15 to 20 minutes can actually make part of the body numb and is an excellent technique for gaining control over pain. You start by learning it in a part of the body where there is no pain, and then later can transfer your skill to areas of pain.
8. Imagine circulating the electrical energy from your brain or your neck down the back of a part of the body as you breathe in, and up the front of that part of the body as you breathe out. This, again, normalizes or balances the normal internal feelings in that part of the body, or if you do it in the body as a whole, in the entire body.
9. Expand the electromagnetic energy field around the body. Electricity creates magnetism. Thus, if you create a 1 inch (2.5 cm) and then a 12 inch (30 cm) halo of electromagnetic energy around any part of the body, or the body as a whole, it brings that part of the body into balance and gives you control over feelings.

During the days that follow, you will have an opportunity to practise/experience each of these.

Once you have gained control over these natural body feelings, then you carry out the same practice when there is an *emotional* tension.

Ultimately, you have only a limited number of solutions to major psychological distress. This includes asserting yourself or fighting back to change the situation, divorcing unacceptable situations with joy, or accepting and forgiving. It is not a question of right or wrong, it is a question of which *feels* best. Ultimately, you can learn to base decisions upon feelings. The process is not easy, and requires discipline and practice, but it is exquisitely simple.

Evaluating Stress

Now you're ready to evaluate some aspects of stress in your life. Firstly, you need to look at any 'unfinished business' by asking yourself the following questions.

1. Do you have significant unfinished business with:
   a. any member of your family?
   b. any friend or colleague?
   c. any teacher or any other person in your life?
   d. any aspect of religion?
   e. any aspect of authority?
   f. any aspect of government?
   g. any aspect of education?
2. Overall, how victimized do you feel?
3. How well-adjusted do you feel sexually?
4. Do you feel sexually adequate?
5. Do you feel financially vulnerable?
6. Do you have problems accepting responsibility?
7. Do you have resentment when someone else has failed to take responsibility?
8. Overall, how disappointed do you feel in life?
9. How strong is your self-esteem?
10. How judgemental are you?
11. How forgiving are you?
12. How capable are you of expressing to friends and family your personal needs and desires?
13. How strong is your personal belief in a divine power or God?
14. How strong is your personal belief in a soul or the survival of physical life?
15. How strong is you personal belief in the 'golden rule' (see page 8)?

As you go through your daily routine, your daily adjustment, or your daily exercises, these questions will be the dominant themes with which you work, but before you begin this, you might want to take a look at your total life stress by working through the following tests.

These will help to give you an understanding of the most critical stressors in your life. You can spend some extra time dealing with those stressors as you carry out your 90-day programme.

PERSONAL STRESS ASSESSMENT

Total Life Stress Test

Name   **Date**

Circle the answers appropriate for you.

I. Chemical Stress

A. *Dietary Stress*
Average daily sugar consumption   (*total used*)

Sugar added to food or drink (teaspoons)	0 1 2 3 4
Bun, piece of pie/cake, other dessert (no. per day)	0 1 2 3 4
Coke or can of fizzy drink, chocolate bar (no. per day)	0 1 2 3 4
Banana split, commercial milk shake, sundae etc (no. per day)	0 1 2 3 4
White flour (white bread, spaghetti etc) (circle 2 if you use it)	2

Average daily salt consumption

I add salt to my food	0 1 2 3 4
I eat salty food	0 1 2 3 4

Average daily caffeine consumption (0 = none; 4 = 4 or more/day)

Coffee (1 point per cup)	0 1 2 3 4
Tea (1 point per cup)	0 1 2 3 4
Cola drink (1 point per glass)	0 1 2 3 4
Caffeine tables (1 point each)	0 1 2 3 4

Dietary Subtotal

B. *Other Chemical Stress*
(Circle the number by each statement that applies)

Drinking water

Your water is chlorinated	1
Your water is fluoridated	2

20

Soil and air pollution

Live within 10 miles of city of 500,000 or more	4
Live within 10 miles of city of 250,000 or more	2
Live within 10 miles of city of 50,000 or more	2
Live in the country but pesticides, herbicides, and/or chemical fertilizer used	4
Exposed to cigarette smoke of someone else more than 1 hour per day	4

Drugs (for any amount of usage, circle 4)

Antidepressants	4
Tranquillizers	4
Sleeping pills	4
Narcotics	4
Other pain relievers	4
Marijuana or other illegal drugs	4

Drug Subtotal

Nicotine (circle those that apply)

3–10 cigarettes per day	4
11–20 cigarettes per day	8
21–30 cigarettes per day	10
31–40 cigarettes per day	20
Over 40 cigarettes per day	40
I smoke cigars	4
I smoke a pipe	4
I use chewing tobacco	8

Nicotine Subtotal

Average daily alcohol consumption

1 drink = 1 measure of spirits; or 1 pint beer; or 1 glass of wine

1 drink per day	2
2 drinks per day	4
3 or more drinks per day	20

Alcohol Subtotal

II. Physical Stress

Weight (circle that which applies)

Underweight more than 10lb	5
10–15lb overweight	5
16–25lb overweight	10

| 26–40lb overweight | 20 |
| More than 40lb overweight | 40 |

Activity (circle that which applies)

Adequate exercise = doubling heartbeat and/or sweating a minimum of 30 minutes per workout

Adequate exercise 3 days or more per week	0
Some physical exercise 1 or 2 days per week	15
No regular exercise	40

Work stress (circle that which applies)

Sit most of the day	3
Industrial/factory worker	3
Overnight travel more than once a week	5
Work more than 50 hours per week	10
Work varying shifts	10
Work night shift	5
Heavy labour – physically fit	0
Heavy labour – not physically fit	40

Physical Stress Subtotal

III. Attitudinal Stress

A. Holmes-Rahe Social Readjustment Rating
(Circle those events listed below which you have experienced during the past 12 months.)

Death of a spouse	10
Divorce	7
Marital separation	6
Prison term	6
Death of a close family member	5
Personal injury or illness	5
Marriage	5
Fired at work	5
Marital reconciliation	5
Retirement	5
Change in health of family member	4
Pregnancy	4
Sexual difficulties	4
Gain of new family member	4
Business readjustment	4

Change in financial state	4
Death of a close friend	4
Change to different line of work	4
Change in number of arguments with spouse	4
Housing costs over 40% of income	3
Foreclosure of mortgage or borrowing	3
Change in responsibilities at work	3
Son or daughter leaving home	3
Trouble with in-laws	3
Outstanding personal achievement	2
Spouse begins or stops work	3
Begin or end school	3
Change in living conditions	3
Revision of personal habits	2
Trouble with boss	3
Change in work hours or conditions	2
Change in residence	2
Change in schools	2
Change in recreation	2
Change in church activities	2
Change in social activities	2
Housing costs over 25% of income	1
Change in sleeping habits	2
Change in eating habits	1
Vacation, especially if away from home	1
Christmas, or other major holiday	1
Minor violations of the law	1

Total points?

B. *Other Emotional Stress* (circle those that apply)
Sleep

Less than 7 hours per night	4
Usually 7–8 hours per night	0
More than 8 hours per night	2

Relaxation

Relax only during sleep	4
Relax or meditate at least 20 minutes per day	0

Frustration at work

Enjoy work	0
Mildly frustrated by job	1
Moderately frustrated by job	4

Very frustrated by job	8
Lack of authority at job	8
Boss doesn't trust me	8

Marital status

Married, happily	0
Married, moderately unhappy	4
Married, very unhappy	8
Unmarried man over 30	2
Unmarried woman over 30	1

Usual mood

Happy, well adjusted	0
Moderately angry, depressed or frustrated	4
Very angry, depressed, or frustrated	8

Overall attitude

Degree of feeling of hopelessness	0 1 2 3 4
Degree of feeling depressed	0 1 2 3 4
Inability to achieve major goal	0 1 2 3 4
Inability to achieve close love/intimacy	0 1 2 3 4
Degree to which I am frustrated, annoyed, and/or angry because someone attacked or harmed me or prevented me from happiness	0 1 2 3 4

(Below, score a 0 if you agree; score a 1, 2, 3, or 4 if you disagree.)

Satisfied and in control of my life	0 1 2 3 4
Experience happiness regularly	0 1 2 3 4
Believe I am responsible for my happiness	0 1 2 3 4
Believe and experience happiness is an inside job	0 1 2 3 4

Any other major emotional stress not mentioned above.
You judge intensity 0–10

Other Emotional Stress Subtotal
Attitudinal Stress Subtotal

Total Life Stress

I. Chemical Total
II. Physical Total
III. Attitudinal Total

Total Life Stress Total

Scoring and Goal Setting

Dietary Subtotal
For a score above 10, read the nutritional section several times.

Drug Subtotal
For a score of 4 or more, you need this programme!

Nicotine
For *any score*, you need this programme. Plan to give up completely by Day 30.

Alcohol
For a score above 6, you need this programme. Plan to give up completely by Day 30.

Physical Stress Subtotal
For a score of 40 or more, read the physical exercise section several times.

Social Readjustment Rating
For a score of 30 or more, you need this programme.

Other Emotional Stress
For a score of 10 or more, you'll benefit from this programme.

List here your most important Goals

(The first nine statements are adapted from an article that appeared in *Natural Health*, January/February 1992. The other statements round it out with other aspects I consider essential.)

Grade yourself on a scale of 0 (none) to 10 (most possible) for each statement.

1. My sense of meaning/purpose in my life (work, family, relationships, activities).
2. My ability to express anger appropriately to defend myself.
3. My ability to ask friends and family for support when I feel lonely or troubled.
4. My ability to ask friends or family for favours.
5. My ability to say 'no' when someone asks for a favour I cannot or don't wish to do.
6. The degree to which I fulfil my personal concept of a healthy lifestyle (diet, exercise, relaxation).
7. The degree to which I fulfil my need to play.
8. The degree to which I am free of depression.
9. My freedom from fulfilling a prescribed role in my life (wife, husband, parent, boss, the 'right' thing to do) to the exclusion of my own needs.
10. My overall happiness.
11. The degree to which I feel autonomous – responsible for my own happiness. (No one else can make me happy or deprive me of my happiness.)
12. The degree to which I am free of the need to 'find the right person' to fulfil my needs/desires.
13. The degree to which I am free of blaming anyone else for my problems.
14. The degree to which I am free of being a victim.
15. My self-esteem.
16. My ability to receive and give love/nurturing.
17. My ability to express my needs and desires.
18. My ability to accept responsibility for solving my problems and using problems as an opportunity for growth.
19. My overall satisfaction with my sexuality and sexual life.
20. My sense of spirituality.
21. My overall health.

Scoring

If you score less than 7 on any statement or less than 150 overall, your health and immune system are at risk. Take responsibility for improving these crucial aspects of life. The self-healing programme is definitely for you.

Now ask yourself: Is my health worthwhile to me? Am I willing to put effort into feeling better and more energetic?

90 Days to Stress-free Living offers you an opportunity to *treat* yourself to a healthy lifestyle. Although it requres time – at least one hour per day – you deserve it. And you *will* feel better if you follow it.

Please note that you'll sometimes be asked to visualize. 'Visualization' is the normal way you use your mind. Every word you think is automatically converted into the appropriate image or vision. 'Seeing' means an internal image or awareness of knowing. Your mind knows how to image. As you read and do the daily exercises, you will understand more and more how to use this skill to best advantage.

Now you are ready to begin your 90-day programme.

Day 1

Begin with 2 or 3 repetitions of the 5 limbering exercises, plus 3 sit-ups.

Exercise

Choose your favourite exercise mode and enjoy it.

Relaxation and Body Balancing

Read twice and then do.

For the first 3 minutes, relax and balance your body.

For the next 2 minutes repeat the power word for today: *sacred.*

You have a body – a magnificent temple in which you live. Reflect upon the complexity, the uniqueness, the beauty, the sacredness of your body.

Feel Good to Yourself
LOVE YOUR BODY

Feel good to yourself by loving your body. Whatever you have as a body, remember it is the holy temple in which you live. Most problems of the body are the result of lifestyle. So, if you don't like your body, change your lifestyle. Clean up your habits, eat right and exercise adequately. Think right, think positively.

You can change your weight, posture, endurance, strength, and fitness. Above all, you can train yourself to smile – outwardly and inwardly. If you smile favourably upon your body, you are only appreciating God's work.

No child can thrive without nurturing and love. Nurture and love your body – each moment of each day.

Rejoice in the beauty and wisdom of your body and feel good.

Day 2

Practise 3 repetitions of each of the 5 limbering exercises plus 3 sit-ups.

Exercise

Choose your exercise mode and enjoy it.

Relaxation and Body Balancing

Read twice and then do.

For the first 3 minutes, relax and balance your body.

For the next 2 minutes repeat the power word for today: *bless*.

I have a mind – a marvellous, intelligent mind which helps me learn and experience the world. I appreciate and honour the unique ability of my mind to understand the universe and myself.

Feel Good to Yourself
WHO ARE YOU?

Feel good to yourself by examining who you are. Tune in to your mind and ask yourself these questions:

* Am I my thinking? Does every thought I have reflect the best of myself?

* Do the facts I have stored and remember represent the real me?

* Am I mathematics or English? Geography or history? Am I images of everything I've experienced?

- Is it my *mind* that survives death – or is it my consciousness, my awareness?

Repeat to yourself and feel the meaning of these statements: 'I have a mind, a powerful, intelligent mind. I love my mind for it allows me to learn and to experience life.'

Feel good to yourself by saying, 'I have a mind, and I am much more than my mind. I *direct* my mind to focus its attention.'

Day 3

Do 4 repetitions of each of the 5 limbering exercises and 4 sit-ups.

If adding one repetition each day is not comfortable, add one repetition every third to fifth day, but keep at it.

Exercise

Choose your exercise mode and enjoy it.

Relaxation

Relaxation is the state of body and mind entered when you focus your attention on any thought which is not stressful.

Spend 10 minutes just observing your breathing. *Feel* yourself breathe. Concentrate upon breathing deep into your abdomen, filling your lungs from the bottom up.

Just observe your mind and feelings as you breathe. Be aware of the idle chatter of your mind.

Ideally you will repeat this exercise later today. Begin to establish a habit of doing your special mental programme twice daily at the same times each day. Gradually you will move to 15 minutes twice a day.

You deserve to have 30 minutes of good-quality, personal time each day. You will be more productive and more effective if you do.

BREATH

Another great feel good technique is to learn to imagine you are using your breath to collect tension and release it.

Do it systematically.

Breathe in and collect tension from your feet and legs, breathe out and release it.

Breathe in and collect tension in your back, abdomen and pelvis; breathe out and release it.

Breathe in, collect tension in your chest, breathe out and let it go.

Breathe in, collect tension in your arms, neck, and face; breathe out and release it. Doing it this way you can relax your entire body in one minute.

Day 4

Practise 5 repetitions of each of the 5 limbering exercises plus 5 sit-ups.

Exercise

Choose your exercise mode and enjoy it.

Relaxation

Today spend 10 minutes (twice) focusing on these words:

'I am . . .' as you breathe in,

'. . . relaxed' as you breathe out.
Just continue repeating the words and be aware of your sensations as you experience ever deepening states of relaxation.

Feel Good to Yourself
RELAXATION

Relaxation is one of the best feel good techniques. It takes far less energy to relax than to hold yourself tense.

Relaxation can be assisted by focusing on *any* non-stressful thought. Words, images, sounds, or music can all help you to relax deeply.

Practise relaxation 20 minutes twice a day, and you can lower adrenalin production by 50 per cent for the entire 24 hour period.

Although you should not practise deep relaxation while driving, regular relaxation practice during the day will allow you to arrive at your destination with more energy.

A simple, effective way to begin relaxation is to assume a comfortable position, close your eyes, and repeat to yourself, 'I am . . .' as you breathe in, '. . . relaxed' as you breathe out. This technique will lead to deep relaxation in most people within 10 minutes.

Day 5

Practise 6 repetitions of each of the 5 limbering exercises plus 6 sit-ups.

Exercise

Choose your exercise mode and enjoy it.

Relaxation

Today concentrate in each 10 minute session upon just feeling systematically the feedback from your scalp, head, face, neck, throat, arms and hands, chest and breasts, abdomen, lower back, buttocks, pelvis, sexual organs, legs and feet.

As you feel, consciously let go of the tension in each area. Repeat several times until you experience real relaxation. And note the changing sensations as you focus on any one area.

Feel Good to Yourself
FEELING PULSES

Learning to feel the blood flowing through your body is a marvellous feel good approach.

Sense and feel for the pulse of your heartbeat in your hands. Once you learn this, feel the pulse in your heart itself, then in your abdomen, feet and legs, and finally in your lips and neck and throat.

There is only one place in the body where you should avoid feeling the pulse – inside your head. If you ever feel a pulse there, switch to your hand. And notice the warmth and pleasant feelings of life flowing into your body.

Feel good by pulsing.

Day 6

Practise 7 repetitions of each of the 5 limbering exercises plus 7 sit-ups.

Exercise

Choose your exercise mode and enjoy it.

Relaxation/Concentration

Focus in each 10 minute exercise upon observing your thumb. Just examine it. Keep your attention as focused upon your thumb as possible. After 5 minutes, close your eyes and continue to see your thumb. Feel it. Concentrate until at least 95 per cent of your entire awareness is upon your thumb.

Before you return to your normal state of awareness, do a quick survey of your entire body. Be aware of any area of tension and let go!

Feel Good to Yourself
FRUIT

Feel good to yourself by becoming intimately aware of your favourite fruit. Select a luscious, fully ripe piece of fruit and examine it carefully. Examine the colour and texture, the shape and size, the delightful smell. Savour the thought of tasting your fruit. Notice whether your saliva is flowing in anticipation.

Slowly peel your fruit, taking time to appreciate the feel, the odour, the sound, the image, and finally the taste. As you enjoy each bit of your fruit, sense how it will become part of your body. Feel it pleasantly pleasing your stomach, nourishing every cell of your body.

Can you imagine how it feels to be that piece of fruit?

Feel good to yourself by being aware of your dependence upon many different foods to nourish and please you.

Day 7

Practise 8 repetitions of each of the 5 limbering exercises plus 8 sit-ups.

Exercise

Choose your exercise mode and enjoy it.

Relaxation and Body Balancing

Today focus upon really loving and appreciating each part of your body. Sense, see, feel, and appreciate the wonderful miracle of each part systematically. Don't skimp! Desire to do good to your body.

Before you return to your normal state of awareness, do a quick survey of your entire body. Be aware of any area of tension and let go!

Feel Good to Yourself
THE BODY BEAUTIFUL

Feel good to yourself by living the reality of the body beautiful. Recognize the sanctity of the temple in which you live, loving it and treating it with the respect you know it deserves.

Recognize that every atom of every cell in every organ of your body is part of the divine creation.

Be aware that when you invite divine love into every beat of your heart you are creating abundant energy to enhance health.

Know that your habits, your eating, your exercise, and especially your thinking release that potential for perfect health.

Charge your body, mind, and emotions with the ideals of your inner self. Fill your life with the sacred energy by attunement with your spiritual ideals and you'll reap the rewards of feeling good.

Day 8

Practise 9 repetitions of each of the 5 limbering exercises plus 9 sit-ups.

Exercise

Choose your exercise mode for today and enjoy it.

Relaxation

Read this twice then practise it.

Once you are in a comfortable position, imagine breathing in and out through the skin of your feet. You may imagine the air simply coming in and out, like a bellows. Or you may imagine the air entering your feet, travelling through your legs and abdomen to your lungs as you breathe in; then you breathe out with the air travelling back through your abdomen, and legs, and out through your feet.

Systematically breathe in and out at least two complete breaths through your legs, pelvis, abdomen, chest, arms and hands, neck, and face/skull, and body as a whole.

Before you return to your normal state of awareness, do a quick survey of your entire body. Be aware of any area of tension and let go!

This exercise is particularly good for pain control. Once you learn to do this technique well in a normal, non-painful part of the body, by concentrating your breathing through an area of discomfort for 15 to 20 minutes, that area will become numb or anaesthetized.

Feel Good to Yourself
BREATHING

Breathing is so simple and so important for good health. 'The Breath of Life' – how true that is. Take some deep, slow breaths while I tell you this true story.

A woman came to me one day. She couldn't understand why she felt so tense. 'I exercise regularly', she said. I asked her to do some exercise for me over several minutes. Suddenly, I was sure I knew the answer. I asked her to stop her exercise pattern and simply to stand and breathe slowly and deeply, breathing in to the count of 10 and out to the count of 13. Right there before me, her body began to release its tension. She looked puzzled, 'What is happening?' she asked. 'I feel so much better.' 'In all the years you have been exercising,' I explained, 'you have forgotten to breathe and so the tissues can't breathe either. When you don't breathe, the body becomes tense, the cells unable to get oxygen or to release their waste products through the exhaled air.' I asked the woman to repeat her exercise pattern, now breathing deeply and regularly. She smiled, 'What a gift I have received today. I feel so relaxed.'

Breathing . . . so simple, so important, so relaxing!

Day 9

Practise 10 repetitions of each of the 5 limbering exercises and 10 sit-ups.

Today is a day to enjoy resting from aerobics.

Relaxation

Read twice and then do it.

As you breathe in, imagine you are collecting all tension in your feet; as you breathe out, release the tension. Repeat collecting and releasing at least twice from each area of the body: feet; legs; pelvis; genitalia; abdomen; lower back; chest; shoulders, arms, and hands; neck; face and skull; body as a whole.

Before you return to your normal state of awareness, do a quick survey of your entire body. Be aware of any area of tension and let go!

Feel Good to Yourself
CALM AND SERENE

Remaining calm and poised is one key to feeling good. Just as the ocean becomes turbulent during a storm, mental storms such as unfocused anxiety create restless, useless frenzy.

Ultimately, the only sure way to be calm and serene is to practise consistently day after day, hour after hour.

Ideally, you will put yourself in a quiet place, uncross your arms and legs, and repeat as you breathe in 'calm . . .' and as you breathe out '. . . serene.' Practise quietly 15 minutes twice a day as well as consistently throughout the day, reminding yourself once or twice an hour, 'calm . . . serene'.

Over a three month period, your entire being will be much more calm and serene, and you will feel good, recognizing the results of your effort.

Day 10

Practise 11 repetitions of each of the 5 limbering exercises plus 11 sit-ups.

Exercise

Choose your exercise mode and enjoy it.

Body Balancing

Read this twice and then do it.

Be aware that the body is a remarkable electrical device. Imagine that you are circulating that electrical energy. As you breathe in, circulate electrical energy from your heels up the back of your legs, buttocks, back, chest, arms and hands, neck and scalp. As you breathe out, circulate the electrical energy down over the front of your face, hands, arms, neck, chest, abdomen, groin, legs, and feet, into the soles of your feet. Continue circulating the energy until it flows freely through all parts.

Before you return to your normal state of awareness, do a quick survey of your entire body. Be aware of any area of tension and let go!

Feel Good to Yourself
THE ENERGY OF CONNECTEDNESS

Feel good to yourself by focusing intently upon any object. Select an object familiar to you. Note its shape and how the various parts fit together. Can you imagine the inside of the object? Can you sense your object at a microscopic level? Can you sense the individual molecules and atoms that somehow stay together to create the physical 'reality' you observe? How do those atoms differ from those that make up your body? Can you sense the electromagnetic field of the electrons whirling around inside the object you are observing? Is there any connection between your electromagnetic energy and that of your object?

Is there any connection between your electromagnetic energy field and that of other people near you? What is the energy of connectedness?

Feel good to yourself by being connected.

Day 11

Practise 12 repetitions of each of the 5 limbering exercises plus 12 sit-ups.

Exercise

Choose your favourite exercise mode and enjoy it.

Body Balancing

Read this twice and then do it.

Be aware that electricity creates magnetism. Imagine that you are expanding the electromagnetic energy field 1 inch (2.5 cm) around your feet. Then allow this expanded energy to flow around your ankles, calves, knees, thighs, groin, buttocks, abdomen, back, chest, shoulders, arms, hands, neck, face, and scalp.

Then repeat, systematically, expanding the electromagnetic energy field by 12 inches (30 cm) around your feet, ankles, calves, knees, thighs, groin, buttocks, abdomen, back, chest, shoulders, arms, hands, neck, face, and scalp.

This is another excellent technique for controlling pain. It is impossible to feel pain in any part of the body when you are surrounded by 12 inches of electromagnetic energy.

This technique is also useful for 'out of body' experiences.

In the state of 12 inch expansion, individuals may feel as if the body is asleep and the mind is alert. Sometimes you feel as if you arc floating in space.

Before ending this session, imagine that the 12 inch halo is filled with a golden orange light. Then allow the 12 inches of golden orange light to flow back into each part of your body, re-energizing and rejuvenating every cell in your body.

Feel Good to Yourself
EXPLORE YOUR INNER SELF

Feel good to yourself by exploring your inner resources. Recognize your limitless reservoir of thoughts; your inner source of lofty spiritual aspirations and ideals.

Sense your deep reserves of sympathy and compassion. Touch your fountains of enthusiasm. Be aware of the endless rivers of intuitive creativity available to you.

The sun of happiness burns within your heart. Feast upon your inner faith in the purpose of life. Find meaning in the beauty of contemplation upon your ideals.

Recognize that your soul is the essence of happiness. Joy, peace, calmness, and serenity are the fruits of reflection.

Know that in every cloud there is an opportunity to find the silver lining, the rainbow after the storm.

Feel good to yourself by experiencing the rich depth of your inner self.

Day 12

Practise 13 repetitions of each of the 5 limbering exercises plus 13 sit-ups.

Exercise

Choose your exercise mode for today and enjoy it.

Body Balancing

Read this twice and do it.

After you have placed yourself into a state of relaxation, create an image of a circular dial with the numbers 0 to 10 and a single hand. Imagine that this dial represents your level of stress. Note where your stress level is. Then move the hand to zero. Do not worry about where you *feel* your stress level is; just move the stress dial to zero and hold it there.

Concentrate for at least 10 minutes keeping the stress dial at zero. Then get the feedback from your body and determine how closely your body follows your image of zero stress. The more you practise, the greater will become your ability to turn your stress level to zero.

Feel Good to Yourself
CREATING DESIRED CONDITIONS

Can you focus entirely upon creating the condition desired? Instead of eliminating an undesired condition, can you seek a solution that creates the *desired* result?

For instance, if you desire a specific weight, instead of focusing on *losing* weight, use words and images which create the ideal weight.

The same is true for *every* aspect of life, from wealth to sports. *Think and Grow Rich* and *The Inner Game of Tennis* provide good discussion of positive creative thinking and visualization. Whatever your goals in life, to feel good, focus your attention upon *creating* the condition desired.

Day 13

Practise 14 repetitions of each of the 5 limbering exercises and 14 sit-ups.

Exercise

Choose your exercise mode and enjoy it.

Relaxation and Body Balancing

Memorize the following phrases:

> My arms and legs are heavy and warm
> My heartbeat is calm and regular
> My breathing is free and easy
> My abdomen is warm
> My forehead is cool
> My mind is quiet and still.

Once memorized, repeat each phrase 3 to 5 times, repeating to yourself the first half of each phrase while breathing in, the second half while breathing out.

Once you've learned this sequence, you may reinforce the effect by creating images to enhance the meaning of the words.

Feel Good to Yourself
POSITIVE THOUGHTS AND IMAGES

To feel really good, dedicate one day each week to focusing *only* upon *positive* thoughts and images.

Set yourself up the night before by writing out several positive affirmations. When you awaken, repeat the affirmations to yourself for at least 10 minutes. As you do so, contemplate the meaning of these phrases.

Whenever you find yourself shifting attention to any negative thoughts, ask yourself how that relates to the affirmations you've chosen for the day.

Explore solutions to the perceived problem. How do you *create the opposite*?

After a few weeks, you may want to spend every day focusing only on positive thoughts.

Day 14

Practise 15 repetitions of each of the 5 limbering exercises and 15 sit-ups.

Exercise

Choose your exercise mode for today and enjoy it.

Body Balancing

Now is the time to determine which relaxation/body balancing technique of the past days works best for you. If in doubt, keep reviewing the different techniques until your body's sensory feedback tells you unequivocally which technique leads you to optimal relaxation and a feeling of balance in *each* part of your body.

Every day henceforth, the first three minutes of your mental programme will be devoted to relaxing and balancing your body.

The next two minutes you will focus on repeating your *power word* of the day, saying it as you breathe in and as you breathe out. Move your lips. It helps you concentrate and focus your mind. Each day you will concentrate on a different power word. *Each day, then:*

1. Read the exercise twice
2. Relax and balance body tension (3 minutes)
3. Breathe and say your power word (2 minutes)
4. Do the contemplation or insight exercise (10 minutes)
5. The remaining 10 minutes of each session will be aimed at emotional or spiritual integration.

Feel Good to Yourself
LEARNING SOMETHING NEW

A really powerful feel good technique is to learn something new each day.

Whenever you hear or read a word or phrase you don't know, look it up. It takes only a minute or two, but in a few years, you can double your usual vocabulary.

Make learning the fun experience it is for young children. We can all take a lesson from the enthusiasm of toddlers in learning new words and having new experiences.

One of the best ways to avoid boredom is to concentrate upon learning. Do you really know what 'supercalfaciferous' means? It's a fun word to begin learning.

Day 15

Practise 16 repetitions of each of the 5 limbering exercises and 16 sit-ups.

Exercise

Choose your exercise mode and enjoy it.

Relaxation and Body Balancing

For the first three minutes, relax and balance your body.

For the next two minutes repeat the power word.

Today's word is *feel*.

Then recall the *worst* trauma/pain (physical or emotional) of your life.

Re-experience the *feeling*. Note where you feel and what you feel.

Then let go.

Repeat several times.

The purpose of this exercise is learning to detach even if you can't solve the problem.

Feel Good to Yourself
PROBLEMS

A healthy way to deal with problems is to look at them as opportunities for growth. For instance, whenever a real crisis arises, ask yourself: What did I do to contribute to this situation? What can I learn from the situation so that I won't have to experience such a problem again?

The possible lessons are many: patience, wisdom, forgiveness, tolerance, serenity, and many others. The basic message is: when life gives you lemons, learn to make lemonade. Put a little bit of honey into your life by seeing the good.

Day 16

Practise 17 repetitions of each of the 5 limbering exercises plus 17 sit-ups.

Today is a day to enjoy resting.

Relaxation and Body Balancing

For the first 3 minutes, relax and balance your body.

Then repeat the power words for the next 2 minutes.

Today's power words are: *let go*.

Now once again recall the worst trauma/pain of your life.

Re-experience the feeling. Then ask yourself: how much energy am I devoting to this old problem every day?

Feel the answer. Then *let go*.

Repeat several times.

Feel Good to Yourself
MIND STORMING

Mind storming is a unique, personal way to feel good. All it requires is a pad and paper, and you.

Start by asking one special very important question at the top of a page.

Then write as many answers as you can, aiming for a minimum of 20. Write down every possibility that comes to mind, no matter how wild or far out it seems.

Set a time period for the answers, say 10 to at the most 20 minutes. Avoid criticizing or judging any answer. Just put down any possible solution. Making a list spontaneously and without judgment can be very helpful.

When all the possible solutions are on paper, then grade each one on a scale of 0 to 10 as to ease or likelihood.

Mind storming may provide the best solution to your problems and help you feel good.

Day 17

Practise 18 repetitions of each of the 5 limbering exercises plus 18 sit-ups.

Exercise

Choose your favourite mode of exercise and enjoy it.

Relaxation and Body Balancing

For the first 3 minutes, relax and balance your body.

For the next 2 minutes, repeat the power word.

Today's power word is *assert*.

Now once again recall the worst trauma/pain of your life.

Re-experience the feeling. Then ask yourself: am I *ready* to deal with all unfinished aspects of that problem? Feel the answer.

Can I/should I assert myself to convince the person responsible for my pain to acknowledge my hurt?

Would I feel satisfied if they apologized? If they won't apologize, am I willing to detach?

Feel the answers and let go.

Feel Good to Yourself
PERSONAL POWER

Feeling good is the result of a wise use of power. Power begins with recognition of your inner ability to take charge of most events, knowing that you have the power to choose your attitude towards those aspects you cannot change. Power is the way you treat other people – with respect and dignity, even if you disagree with them.

Power is the attitude you create in your body, your face and your speech. It is the result of your respect for your own dignity. Ultimately, power is living the golden rule (see page 8) – towards yourself and towards others – and feeling good because you deserve to feel good when you use power wisely.

Day 18

Practise 19 repetitions of each of the 5 limbering exercises plus 19 sit-ups.

Exercise

Choose your exercise mode and enjoy it.

Relaxation and Body Balancing

For the first 3 minutes, relax and balance your body.

For the next 2 minutes, repeat the power word for today: *joy*.

Now once again recall the worst trauma/pain of your life.

Re-experience the feeling. Then ask yourself: am I *ready* to deal with all unfinished aspects of that problem? Feel the answer.

If I cannot obtain a satisfactory correction/apology, can I divorce the situation, with joy?

Feel the answer.

Let go.

Repeat several times.

Feel Good to Yourself
RESOLVE ANGER, FEAR, GUILT

Feel good to yourself by resolving unfinished business. Recall any significant past hurt – anger, fear, guilt. Be aware of how it feels. Note exactly where you feel the stress. And ask yourself these questions:

- Is there anything I can do now to correct the situation?

- Can I discuss the hurt with the person responsible and ask them to apologize? Can I sue them?

- Have I found a way to avoid ever having such a problem again?

- What did I learn from that problem that makes me a better person?

- Am I willing to accept and forgive the person(s) involved?

- If not, what will it take for me to forgive?

- Does it make me feel good to hold a grudge?

- Can it solve the problem if I continue to be upset?

- Am I willing to resolve my anger, fear, or guilt in order to feel good?

Day 19

Practise 20 repetitions of each of the 5 limbering exercises plus 20 sit-ups.

Exercise

Choose your exercise mode and enjoy it.

Relaxation and Body Balancing

Read twice and then do.

For the first 3 minutes, relax and balance your body.

For the next 2 minutes, repeat the power word for today: *accept.*

Now once again recall the worst trauma/pain of your life.

Re-experience the feeling. Then ask yourself: am I *ready* to deal with all unfinished aspects of that problem? Feel the answer.

If I cannot obtain a satisfactory correction/apology and cannot or will not divorce with joy, am I willing to accept and forgive? Not to *condone* or approve, but just to accept and forgive?

Feel the answer and let go.

Repeat several times.

COUNSELLING YOURSELF

Feel good to yourself by being your own best counsellor. Most of us give excellent advice to our friends when they ask for our opinion. Do you treat yourself as well as you treat friends and acquaintances?

Is your advice to yourself wise, compassionate, reasonable? If someone approached you with similar problems, how would you advise them to behave?

Whatever your problem, remember it's no different from anyone else's. You have *only* three solutions:

1. *Fight*. Assert yourself through words, actions or the law.

2. *Flight*. Divorce the unacceptable and intolerable with joy.

3. *Go for sainthood*. Accept and forgive that which cannot be changed.

Feel good to yourself by doing good to yourself with wise counselling.

Day 20

Practise 21 repetitions of each of the 5 limbering exercises plus 21 sit-ups. You are now at the maximum number of repetitions you need to maintain flexibility. You will continue at this rate for the remainder of the 90 day programme. (Or, if you like, you *can* build to 42 repetitions of each and benefit even more!)

Exercise

Choose your favourite exercise mode and enjoy it.

Relaxation and Body Balancing

Read twice and then do.

For the first 3 minutes, relax and balance your body.

For the next 2 minutes, repeat the power word.

Today's power word is *forgive*.

Now recall the *second* worst trauma/pain (physical or emotional) of your life.

Re-experience the *feeling*. Note where you feel and what you feel.

Then let go.

Repeat several times.

The purpose of this exercise is learning to detach and forgive even if you can't solve the problem.

THE WISDOM OF AGE ·

Feeling good is recognizing the wisdom that comes with age. In some societies, age is a venerable state and the older one becomes, the more prestige one attains.

Be aware of the benefits of maturity. Recognize each day how fortunate you are to have learned how to avoid certain problems, how to solve others, how to cope with more and more of life's challenges. Wisdom is knowing when to be responsible for a given opportunity and when to detach. Wisdom is knowing how to detach from the things you cannot change. Wisdom is the appropriate use of power in all its manifestations. Wisdom is a loving state of feeling good.

Day 21

Practice 21 repetitions of each of the 5 limbering exercises plus 21 sit-ups.

Exercise

Choose your favourite exercise mode and enjoy it.

Relaxation and Body Balancing

Read twice and then do.

For the first 3 minutes, relax and balance your body.

For the next 2 minutes, repeat the power word.

Today's power word is again *forgive*.

Now once again recall the *second* worst trauma/pain of your life.

Re-experience the *feeling*. Note where you feel and what you feel. Then ask yourself: how much energy am I devoting to this old problem every day?

Feel the answer.

Then let go.

Repeat several times.

Feel Good to Yourself
LOVE

Feeling good is love – the desire to do good to yourself and to others.

If you cultivate towards the whole world a state of love, then your life will be fulfilled. Love is the miracle which restores health.

Love is the gift you give to yourself when you help someone else. Whatever you give with a desire to do good is returned many times in the feel good reward.

Any reason is right for giving love, for doing good to others, for forgiving those who have hurt you. Ultimately, love is the supreme feeling good attitude.

Day 22

Practise 21 repetitions of each of the 5 limbering exercises plus 21 sit-ups.

Exercise

Choose your favourite exercise mode and enjoy it.

Relaxation and Body Balancing

Read twice and then do.

For the first 3 minutes, relax and balance your body.

For the next 2 minutes, repeat the power word.

Today's power word is again *forgive*.

Again recall the second worst trauma/pain of your life.

Re-experience the feeling. Then ask yourself: am I *ready* to deal with all unfinished aspects of that problem?

Feel the answer.

Can I/should I assert myself to convince the person responsible for my pain to acknowledge my hurt?

Would I feel satisfied if they apologized? If they won't apologize, am I willing to detach?

Feel the answer.

Then let go.

Feel Good to Yourself
TAKE RISKS

Feel good to yourself by taking risks – not foolish or dangerous risks – but risking the possibility of failing to achieve a specific goal. Set your sights on the highest possible goal and use all your confidence and motivation to meet the challenges of life.

The fun is often in playing the game. Every day you take risks – in breathing, eating, driving, walking. Choose your risks wisely. Use your intuition to help you select the risks worth pursuing.

Actually, you never lose by trying, for you gain new skill, knowledge, courage, and strength when you take responsibility for attempting your dream.

Enjoy the challenge of taking reasonable and wise risks and FGTY knowing you have an opportunity to grow.

Day 23

Practise 21 repetitions of each of the 5 limbering exercises and 21 sit-ups.

Today you can enjoy resting from your aerobic exercise.

Relaxation and Body Balancing

Read twice and then do.

For the first 3 minutes, relax and balance your body.

For the next 2 minutes, repeat the power word for today: *forgive.*

Again recall the second worst trauma/pain of your life.

Re-experience the feeling. Then ask yourself: Am I *ready* to deal with all unfinished aspects of that problem? Feel the answer.

If I cannot obtain a satisfactory correction/apology, can I divorce the situation with joy?

Feel the answer.

Let go.

Repeat several times.

Feel Good to Yourself
CREATE JOY

Feel good to yourself by holding on to every little bubble of joy that appears in your life. Expand it; contemplate it. Meditate on joy. Look not for the limitations of your instance of joy, but nurture it with enthusiasm.

Use the energy of joy to create ever-expanding bubbles of joy in various aspects of your life. Concentrate on joy until your small bubble expands and encloses the ocean of your consciousness.

When you focus upon joy you have no room for fear or sadness. Ask yourself each day: how much joy can I find? Look for joy; create a mental magnet to attract joy; expect joy; and accept it in its many manifestations.

And expand your joy even more by spreading it. Share joy with everyone you meet, especially your family.

FGTY by being an example of joy.

Day 24

Practise 21 repetitions of each of the 5 limbering exercises plus 21 sit-ups.

Exercise

Choose an exercise mode and enjoy it.

Relaxation and Body Balancing

Read twice and then do.

For the first 3 minutes, relax and balance your body.

For the next 2 minutes, repeat the power word.

Today's power word is again *forgive*.

Now again recall the second worst trauma/pain of your life.

Re-experience the feeling. Then ask yourself: am I *ready* to deal with all unfinished aspects of that problem? Feel the answer.

If I cannot obtain a satisfactory correction/ apology and cannot or will not divorce with joy, am I willing to accept and forgive? Not to *condone* or approve, but just to accept and forgive?

Feel the answer and let go.

Repeat several times.

Feel Good to Yourself
GROWTH

Feel good to yourself by understanding 'growth'.

Growth is a combination of knowledge, insight, wisdom, and experience. It is the development of character. Growth is a willingness to change, to explore new concepts and activities, to develop relations. Growth is the response to challenge, the wisdom of seeing obstacles as opportunities, to learn from disappointments.

Without psychological, mental, emotional, and spiritual growth, you are not living but dying. Progress and change may provide controversy and conflict, but they also encourage depth and strength of character.

Individual and spiritual growth are essential for success in all relationships, especially marriage.

FGTY by encouraging yourself to grow – in wisdom and love.

Day 25

Practise 21 repetitions of each of the 5 limbering exercises plus 21 sit-ups.

Exercise

Choose an exercise mode and enjoy it.

Relaxation and Body Balancing

Read twice and then do.

First 3 minutes: relax and balance your body.

For the next 2 minutes repeat the power word.

Today's word is *complete*.

Recall any current *unfinished* business causing you anger, guilt, or depression.

Re-experience the feeling. Note where you feel and what you feel.

Then let go.

Repeat several times. The purpose of this exercise is learning to detach even if you can't solve the problem.

Feel Good to Yourself
HARMONY

Feel good to yourself by exploring the harmony of nature: night and day; the seasons; the relations of plants and animals; the harmonious relationship of colours, each representing a visual frequency gently separating red from orange, yellow, green, blue, indigo, and violet.

Be aware of the harmony of musical notes, representing an audible frequency that separates A from B from C.

Harmony is a representation of rhythm or frequency. Just as there is a rhythm of day and night; spring, summer, autumn, and winter; there is an internal harmony of the body and mind: asleep and awake; rest and action; learning and using.

Feel good to yourself by aligning yourself with your inner harmony.

Day 26

Practise 21 repetitions of each of the 5 limbering exercises plus 21 sit-ups.

Exercise

Choose an exercise mode and enjoy it.

Relaxation and Body Balancing

Read twice and then do.

For the first 3 minutes, relax and balance your body.

For the next 2 minutes, repeat the power word.

Today's power word is *complete*.

Now once again recall any current unfinished business causing you anger, guilt, or depression.

Re-experience the feeling. Note where you feel and what you feel. Then ask yourself: how much energy am I devoting to this old problem every day? Feel the answer. Then let go.

Repeat several times.

Feel Good to Yourself
IMAGERY

Learning to create positive images is a marvellous way to feel good. Ultimately, it is the images we hold in our minds that determine *how* we feel.

Start by closing your eyes and creating an image of your favourite flower; savour it, smell it.

Then create an image of your favourite food. Smell and taste it. Notice your mouth watering.

Now move on to creating an image of your happiest past moments. Once you learn to do this well, begin to picture happy future scenes and solutions to current problems. Feel good by seeing good.

Day 27

Practise 21 repetitions of each of the 5 limbering exercises plus 21 sit-ups.

Exercise

Choose your favourite mode of exercise and enjoy it.

Relaxation and Body Balancing

Read twice and then do.

For the first 3 minutes, relax and balance your body.

For the next 2 minutes, repeat the power word.

Today's power word is *complete*.

Again recall any current unfinished business causing you anger, guilt, or depression.

Re-experience the feeling. Then ask yourself: am I ready to deal with all unfinished aspects of that problem? Feel the answer.

Can I/should I assert myself to convince the person responsible for my pain to acknowledge my hurt?

Would I feel satisfied if they apologized? If they won't apologize, am I willing to detach?

Feel the answers and let go.

Feel Good to Yourself
STRESS

Stress is an unavoidable aspect of life. Indeed, Dr Hans Selye, the great Canadian physician who did the most critical work on stress, actually talks about good stress.

To feel good about stress, remember: most stress is under your control. If you feel treated unfairly, assert yourself calmly and fairly. Learn the broken record approach of Manual Smith from *When I Say No I Feel Guilty*. It's a marvellous way of detaching, being free of anger or emotional stress. Just practise carefully stating your needs and desires in a simple positive fashion. Say the phrases over and over to yourself and then to the person who has offended – or 'stressed' – you. And remember, you control your reactions.

Day 28

Practise 21 repetitions of each of the 5 limbering exercises plus 21 sit-ups.

Exercise

Choose your exercise mode and enjoy it.

Relaxation and Body Balancing

Read twice and then do.

For the first 3 minutes, relax and balance your body.

For the next 2 minutes, repeat the power word for today: *complete*.

Now once again recall any current unfinished business causing you anger, guilt or depression.

Re-experience the feeling. Then ask yourself: am I ready to deal with all unfinished aspects of that problem? Feel the answer.

If I cannot obtain a satisfactory correction/apology, can I divorce the situation with joy?

Feel the answer.

Let go.

Repeat several times.

SAYING NO

To feel good, learn to say no when a request is unreasonable or can't be accomplished in the time allotted.

Saying no can be a positive experience for both you and the other people in your life.

If you can learn to say no without guilt, depression or anxiety, you're well on the way towards being a 'self-actualized' person. You have a *right* to your needs, desires, and priorities, if you are not harming anyone with your decision. Being a doormat for everyone or anyone is not good for you or anyone else.

Practise saying no to unreasonable requests. Do it with a smile and grace, and you'll feel good all day.

Day 29

Practise 21 repetitions of each of the 5 limbering exercises plus 21 sit-ups.

Exercise

Choose your exercise mode and enjoy it.

Relaxation and Body Balancing

Read twice and then do.

For the first 3 minutes, relax and balance your body.

For the next 2 minutes, repeat the power word for today: *complete*.

Again recall any current unfinished business causing you anger, guilt, or depression.

Re-experience the feeling. Then ask yourself: am I ready to deal with all unfinished aspects of that problem? Feel the answer.

If I cannot obtain a satisfactory correction/apology and cannot or will not divorce with joy, am I willing to accept and forgive? Not to condone or approve, but just to accept and forgive?

Feel the answer and let go.

Repeat several times.

Feel Good to Yourself
PEACE

Feeling good is peace towards yourself and others. If you seek harmony with everyone around you, then your life will be fulfilled.

There is no happiness greater than peace. The wise esteem peace above all else. Peace is serenity and detachment from those things you cannot change.

Each of us has an opportunity to practise peace – in our minds and hearts, in our actions and deeds, in our words and behaviour. Peace is the state of feeling good about yourself and others.

Spend 15 minutes each day creating a state of serenity and peace and you will feel good the whole day.

Day 30

Practise 21 repetitions of each of the 5 limbering exercises plus 21 sit-ups.

Today you may enjoy resting from your aerobic exercise.

Relaxation and Body Balancing

Read twice and then do.

For the first 3 minutes, relax and balance your body using your favourite technique.

For the next 2 minutes repeat the power word for today: *change*.

Then see yourself standing in front of a mirror.

Examine your body and see the imperfections in posture, muscle tone, weight.

Are you willing to put forth the effort to change those physical aspects which can be changed to create the best possible body for you?

Know the answer.

Feel Good to Yourself
OBSERVING YOURSELF

Feel good to yourself by really seeing yourself at all levels of your being. Stand quietly in a private room in front of a mirror. Remove your clothes and examine your body carefully. Notice how you stand, how good your posture is. Be aware of your muscle tone, of your weight. Are you too fat, too thin, or just right? Note the colour, texture, and quality of your skin, your hair, your smile. Be aware of how your *mood* affects your body. Recall a stressful event and notice where you tighten up. Recall a sad event and notice how you droop. Relive a joyous experience and reap the visual reward.

Especially be aware of changes in your body which you could make – if you chose. Feel good to yourself by choosing the habits and attitude which are best for you.

Day 31

Practise 21 repetitions of each of the 5 limbering exercises plus 21 sit-ups.

Exercise

Choose your exercise mode and enjoy it.

Relaxation and Body Balancing

Read twice and then do.

For the first 3 minutes, relax and balance your body using your favourite technique.

For the next 2 minutes repeat the power word for today: *tolerant.*

Then see yourself standing in front of a mirror.

See yourself change into the opposite sex. Examine your fears and prejudices related to the male or female sex. Be aware of how your personality is influenced by your sexual stereotypes. Change back to seeing yourself as your sex. Are you willing to be more tolerant?

Feel Good to Yourself
STEREOTYPES

Feel good to yourself by exploring your sexual prejudices. Are women the weaker or stronger sex? Is there *any* activity that is 'woman's work' other than bearing a child?

Be aware that early in this century most secretaries were men; in Russia most physicians are women.

Increasingly, there are trends that are equalizing the numbers of men and women in law, politics, medicine, and many of the fields formerly dominated by men. And some men are staying at home to look after children.

Is there any job which you believe 'belongs' to men or women? Should men and women receive equal pay for the same job? Is there any fairness in treating men and women differently? Can you live the golden rule (see page 8) and treat men and women differently?

Should men and women have different rules of behaviour, dress, language, desires?

FGTY by treating all people with respect.

Day 32

Practise 21 repetitions of each of the 5 limbering exercises plus 21 sit-ups.

Exercise

Choose your exercise mode and enjoy it.

Relaxation and Body Balancing

Read twice and then do.

For the first 3 minutes, relax and balance your body using your favourite technique.

For the next 2 minutes repeat the power word for today: *tolerant.*

Then see yourself standing in front of a mirror.

See yourself change skin colour – white to black or vice versa; or red or yellow.

Get into really seeing yourself become another race.

Examine your fears and prejudices related to skin colour. Be aware of how your personality is influenced by your racial prejudices.

Change back to seeing yourself as your race. Are you willing to be more tolerant?

YOUR ATTITUDE TOWARDS OTHERS

Do you feel good about your attitudes towards all other people? Have you examined *why* you like or dislike certain persons? Have you really examined your prejudices? Why don't you like people who . . . ? Fill in the space with your own prejudices!

Do you have prejudices about sex, race, skin colour, religion? Why?

Are you willing to examine your fears that 'they' may harm you – by taking away your life, health, wealth, love, or moral judgments?

Can you imagine accepting – unconditionally – anyone who poses no harm toward you or your loved ones?

Are you willing to go for one full day tolerating everyone you meet? Can you imagine everyone in the world being tolerant of everyone else? Can you imagine actually desiring to do good to everyone you meet?

Day 33

Practise 21 repetitions of each of the 5 limbering exercises plus 21 sit-ups.

Exercise

Choose your exercise mode and enjoy it.

Relaxation and Body Balancing

Read twice and then do.

For the first 3 minutes, relax and balance your body using your favourite technique.

For the next 2 minutes repeat the power word for today: *forgive*.

Then see yourself standing in front of a mirror.

See the image in your mirror become that of the person you have most feared or hated.

Then sense how much *you* contributed to the conflict between you.

Are you willing to forgive yourself for your part of the conflict?

Are you willing to forgive your worst enemy?

Feel Good to Yourself
TREATING PEOPLE RIGHT

Feeling good is a natural result of treating people right and living with your conscience. As long as you avoid excessive guilt, your conscience is a regular reminder of how you *feel* about your personal behaviour. All you have to be certain of is that you desire to treat other people fairly, that you do not consciously or wilfully harm anyone else. As long as you do not harm, you have nothing to fear. And remember, the only thing we have to fear is fear itself. Think help for others and you will keep a clean, healthy conscience. Treating people right is fun and a reward in itself. It pays great dividends in peace of mind.

Day 34

Practise 21 repetitions of each of the 5 limbering exercises plus 21 sit-ups.

Exercise

Choose your exercise mode and enjoy it.

Relaxation and Body Balancing

Read twice and then do.

For the first 3 minutes, relax and balance your body.

For the next 2 minutes repeat the power word for today: *bless.*

Then sense your total relationship with your mother.

Do you have any unfinished business with your mother?

Are you willing to forgive her for any shortcomings?

Are you willing to bless her for her contributions to your well-being?

Feel Good to Yourself
FAMILY ROOTS

Feel good to yourself by understanding your roots. What are the best traits of your mother? Of your father? Of your siblings?

What are the worst traits of your mother? Of your father? Of your siblings?

How much of *your* personality represents the undesirable traits of your mother? Of your father? Of your siblings?

How much of your behaviour reflects the *best* traits of your mother? Of your father? Of your siblings?

Do you reflect desirable or undesirable behaviours of your grandparents or other relatives?

Can you use the worst traits of your family to create a more successful self?

Can you build upon the best traits of your family?

Feel good to yourself by pruning and cultivating your family roots.

Day 35

Practise 21 repetitions of each of the 5 limbering exercises plus 21 sit-ups.

Exercise

Choose your exercise mode and enjoy it.

Relaxation and Body Balancing

Read twice and then do.

For the first 3 minutes, relax and balance your body.

For the next 2 minutes repeat the power word for today: *nurture*.

Again sense your total relationship with your mother.

When you think of your mother, how nurtured do you feel? As you think of your mother, do you have a desire to do good to her?

Feel Good to Yourself
GIVING

Feeling good is a natural benefit of giving something to someone else. Give not so you will get, but knowing you will receive joy and abundance. Recognize that nature is truly abundant and you deserve abundance. By sharing your abundance.

- just to feel good about helping someone else feel good

- to help someone less fortunate

you are sowing the seeds of abundance and of joy. One of the greatest human attributes is the eagerness to help others.

Each day ask yourself: What can I give to others? It may be a kind word or a compliment; a small gift or a big one.

To feel good, think each day what you can give – and act upon it.

Day 36

Practise 21 repetitions of each of the 5 limbering exercises plus 21 sit-ups.

Exercise

Choose your exercise mode and enjoy it.

Relaxation and Body Balancing

Read twice and then do.

For the first 3 minutes, relax and balance your body.

For the next two 2 minutes repeat the power word for today: *bless*.

Then sense your total relationship with your father.

Do you have any unfinished business with your father?

Are you willing to forgive him for any shortcomings?

Are you willing to bless him for his contributions to your well-being?

Feel Good to Yourself
BLESSINGS

Feel good to yourself by blessing all the people who have made your life more pleasant. Even those individuals who presented you with stress may have given you an opportunity to grow in some way.

Start with your parents and mentally bless them for the many contributions to your well-being. Then think about your siblings, teachers, co-workers, and friends, and bless each of them for providing you with love and support.

Be sure to include your spouse, children, and all the others close to you.

And of course the great scientists and artists, inventors, politicians, and military who have made the world a safer, happier, or more beautiful place.

Perhaps the ultimate FGTY experience is to share with all those dear to you how much you appreciate the blessing they have been to you.

Day 37

Practise 21 repetitions of each of the 5 limbering exercises plus 21 sit-ups.

Today is a day to enjoy resting.

Relaxation and Body Balancing

Read twice and then do.

For the first 3 minutes, relax and balance your body.

For the next 2 minutes repeat the power word for today: *nurture*.

Again sense your total relationship with your father.

When you think of your father, how nurtured do you feel? As you think of your father, do you have a desire to do good to him?

Feel Good to Yourself
SHARE THE JOY

Feel good to yourself by radiating the sunshine of mental joy to all who cross your path. See the darkness of the world's problems fade before the light of your cheer. Burn candles of smiles to ignite the bosoms of the joyless.

Allow your love to spread its laughter into the hearts of all you meet. Share your joyous desire to do good – true love – to plants and flowers, animals and humans alike. Be a beacon of joyous light for all to see.

Scatter the richness of your exuberance through the smiles of your heart, reflected in the depths of your eyes. Allow your innermost magnificence of wisdom and love to be expressed in the language of your body and deeds.

FGTY by spreading joy and happiness.

Day 38

Practise 21 repetitions of each of the 5 limbering exercises plus 21 sit-ups.

Exercise

Choose your exercise mode and enjoy it.

Relaxation and Body Balancing

Read twice and then do.

For the first 3 minutes, relax and balance your body.

For the next 2 two minutes repeat the power word for today: *Bless.*

Then sense your total relationship with your siblings (brothers and/or sisters).

Do you have any unfinished business with your siblings? Are you willing to forgive them for any shortcomings?

Are you willing to bless them for their contributions to your well-being?

Feel Good to Yourself
BLESSING LIFE

Feel good to yourself by blessing your life.

Most of us bless our food and at least occasionally bless someone who has helped us. But do you bless someone's sneeze more often than you bless yourself and your life? When you recognize that you've made an error – a sneeze along life's path – do you bless yourself for learning the lesson?

Do you appreciate, thank and bless – the air, water, food, clothes and shelter you have?

Do you bless the place where you work – your financial livelihood?

Do you bless your parents, grandparents, siblings, and teachers who have given you examples of how to live – to be copied or improved?

Do you bless your spouse and your children for the joy and nurturing they provide?

Each time you bless someone else, remember to appreciate and feel good by blessing yourself.

Day 39

Practise 21 repetitions of each of the 5 limbering exercises plus 21 sit-ups.

Exercise

Choose your exercise mode and enjoy it.

Relaxation and Body Balancing

Read twice and then do.

For the first 3 minutes, relax and balance your body.

For the next 2 minutes repeat the power word for today: *nurture*.

Again sense your total relationship with your siblings.

When you think of your siblings, how nurtured do you feel? As you think of your siblings, do you have a desire to do good to them?

Feel Good to Yourself
TOLERANCE

Tolerance is one of the great feel good attitudes. You don't have to agree with everyone or anyone – but you also don't have to judge them or criticize them or curse them. And you can express your disagreement without *being* disagreeable. You have a right to speak up when someone's behaviour is *potentially harmful* to you or to others, but you don't have a right to insist that everyone agrees with or accepts your beliefs. You may be 'right', but you'll be wrong and intolerant if you call them unholy names and attack them. Treating other people right means accepting them as they are, as long as they are not harming you. After all, variety is the spice of life and tolerance is a great feel good virtue.

Day 40

Practise 21 repetitions of each of the 5 limbering exercises plus 21 sit-ups.

Exercise

Choose your exercise mode and enjoy it.

Relaxation and Body Balancing

Read twice and then do.

For the first 3 minutes, relax and balance your body.

For the next 2 minutes repeat the power word for today: *accept*.

As you recall the first 6 years of your life, how nurtured did you feel? Recall all the unfinished business of the first 6 years of your life.

Are you ready to deal with it?

Can you correct the deficits? Can you divorce them? Or can you accept and forgive?

Feel Good to Yourself
SELF-IMAGE

Feel good to yourself by knowing yourself.

How many of your daily stresses are the result of unfinished business from childhood?

Can you recall the most painful experience of your life? Does it still bother you? How about the second most painful experience? Is it still draining you of energy?

And the third most painful memory? How much time or energy do you spend on these living ghosts of your past?

Can you fight any of them now? Should you speak out? Can you divorce them with joy? What did you learn from each of these painful experiences to make you a stronger, better person? Can you make lemonade out of them?

Are you ready to accept and forgive *forever*? Who suffers if you don't finish those lessons?

Feel good to yourself by dealing with your unfinished business.

Day 41

Practise 21 repetitions of each of the 5 limbering exercises plus 21 sit-ups.

Exercise

Choose your exercise mode and enjoy it.

Relaxation and Body Balancing

Read twice and then do.

For the first 3 minutes, relax and balance your body.

For the next 2 minutes repeat the power word for today: *accept.*

As you recall the years 7 to 12 of your life, how nurtured did you feel? Recall all the unfinished business of these years of your life.

Are you ready to deal with it?

Can you correct the deficits? Can you divorce them? Or can you accept and forgive?

Feel Good to Yourself
SIX SOLUTIONS TO WORRY

Dr Arnold Fox, cardiologist and author of *The Beverly Hills Medical Diet* and several other best-selling books, lists these attributes of worry:

- Worry doesn't work
- Worry is a sign of separation from God

- Worry is negative faith

- Most of our worries are not our own

- Worry keeps us in the problem.

His solutions are:

- Concern – awareness of possible trouble and a thoughtful plan for appropriate action.

- Recognize the ideas and solution God provides.

- Focus on positive faith, focus on *creating* the solution.

- Trust in the other person's ability to succeed.

- Focus upon golden opportunities.

Finally:

- don't worry, be happy.

Lincoln said, 'Most people are about as happy as they make up their minds to be.' Make up your mind to be happy. (These thoughts are reproduced from a small brochure Dr Fox hands out freely to patients, friends, and new acquaintances.)

Day 42

Practise 21 repetitions of each of the 5 limbering exercises plus 21 sit-ups.

Exercise

Choose your exercise mode and enjoy it.

Relaxation and Body Balancing

Read twice and then do.

For the first 3 minutes, relax and balance your body.

For the next 2 minutes repeat the power word for today: *forgive*.

As you recall your years 12 to 18, how nurtured did you feel? Recall all the unfinished business of these years of your life.

Are you ready to deal with it?

Can you correct the deficits? Can you divorce them? Or can you accept and forgive?

Feel Good to Yourself
MAKE LEMONADE

When life gives you lemons, make lemonade.

When life's storms will not subside, strive to fly above them. Resolve the problems there, in the space above the clouds, in the rainbow of life.

You can sweeten the lemons of life by adopting the attitude that each problem is an opportunity for greater expression of your humanity, an opportunity to express good will, to be forgiving and tolerant, to be at peace, to have faith that the purpose is good, to have hope that tomorrow will be better, to find joy in the solution, to be motivated to succeed, to use reason and wisdom in achieving a loving solution.

Day 43

Practise 21 repetitions of each of the 5 limbering exercises plus 21 sit-ups.

Exercise

Choose your exercise mode and enjoy it.

Relaxation and Body Balancing

Read twice and then do.

For the first 3 minutes, relax and balance your body.

For the next 2 minutes repeat the power word for today: *forgive*.

As you recall your years since age 18, how nurtured have you felt? Recall all the unfinished business of these years of your life.

Are you ready to deal with it?

Can you correct the deficits? Can you divorce them? Or can you accept and forgive?

Feel Good to Yourself
PLEASURES PAST

Feel good to yourself by recalling the most happy, joyous experience of your life. Sit quietly with your eyes closed and create the memory in great detail. Recall the exact scene, the time of day, the location, the year. See yourself exactly as you were. See your clothes, their colour and texture. Note the details of your surroundings.

Be aware of any other person or persons with you. Sense, see, feel, hear, smell, taste the experience. Can you remember the words, the sounds?

Exactly what aspects make this memory your most joyous? What did you contribute to the situation to make it so perfect? Can you re-create, in your present life, similar situations?

Feel good to yourself by using the pleasures of your past to influence your present.

Day 44

Practise 21 repetitions of each of the 5 limbering exercises plus 21 sit-ups.

This is a day to enjoy resting.

Relaxation and Body Balancing

Read twice and then do.

For the first 3 minutes, relax and balance your body.

For the next 2 minutes repeat the power word for today: *forgive*.

Is there any unfinished trauma or pain in your life?

Are you ready to deal with it?

Can you correct the deficits? Can you divorce them? Or can you accept and forgive?

Feel Good to Yourself
THOUGHTS

To feel good, *think good*. Every second of the day your immune system responds to your thoughts and mood. Psychoneuroimmunology clearly demonstrates that your white blood cells, lymphocytes, and plasma cells are put on alert – or alarm – if your thoughts are those of fear or anger. And those same cells are clobbered by depression; they are depressed. Ambrose Worrall, one of American's most beloved spiritual healers, in his wonderful essay, said 'Every thought is a Prayer'.

Thinking sets in motion spiritual forces to bring about change in body, mind, environment, companions, hopes, and despairs. We should focus on *thinking about creating* the condition desired – not upon eliminating, but in creating.

Think *right* to feel good.

Day 45

Practise 21 repetitions of each of the 5 limbering exercises plus 21 sit-ups.

Exercise

Choose your exercise mode and enjoy it.

Relaxation and Body Balancing

Read twice and then do.

For the first 3 minutes, relax and balance your body.

For the next 2 minutes repeat the power word for today: *change*.

Recall the unfinished pain or trauma in your life.

Can you recognize that pain is the desire to have things other than as they are? Are you ready to change your attitudes in order to finish any unresolved pain? Do you need to fight (assert), divorce with joy, or go for sainthood (accept and forgive)?

Feel Good to Yourself
CONTROLLING YOUR FEARS

Feel good to yourself by controlling yourself.

Once you are an adult your primary responsibility is to treat yourself well. Although there are sometimes unavoidable conflicts of will, your greatest need is to understand your own needs and desires, to do good to yourself by honouring your personal values.
Compromise is often necessary when you are dealing

with others, but avoid compromising yourself. There are personal unalterable values which only you can understand and set.

Learn to control your reactions so that you can live your values; anger and depression are reactions to fear. Feel good to yourself by controlling your fears in a wise and loving way.

Day 46

Practise 21 repetitions of each of the 5 limbering exercises plus 21 sit-ups.

Exercise

Choose your exercise mode and enjoy it.

Relaxation and Body Balancing

Read twice and then do.

For the first 3 minutes, relax and balance your body.

For the next 2 minutes repeat the power word for today: *forgive*.

On a scale of 0 to 10, how forgiving are you?

Have you forgiven everyone who has harmed or hurt you?

Are you willing to forgive just for self-health?

Feel Good to Yourself
OBSERVING YOURSELF

Can you feel good just by observing your reactions for one day without actually getting *stuck* in those reactions?

Plan to awaken and ask yourself immediately, 'How do I feel?' And no matter what the answer was, ask 'Why?'

Think and observe. Just for one day detach and do not judge yourself or others.

Can you understand yourself without taking time to ask where you developed your attitudes? You may be surprised to learn that your irritations or annoyances are primarily with yourself – not with someone else!

Can you allow yourself one day without condemning your thoughts or actions? Just observing and reflecting? You may learn to be more tolerant and forgiving – of both yourself and others.

Day 47

Practise 21 repetitions of each of the 5 limbering exercises plus 21 sit-ups.

Exercise

Choose your exercise mode and enjoy it.

Relaxation and Body Balancing

Read twice and then do.

For the first 3 minutes, relax and balance your body.

For the next 2 minutes repeat the power word for today: *love*.

On a scale of 0 to 10, how loving are you?

Feel Good to Yourself
LOVE

Feel good to yourself with an understanding of love. Love is the essence of life and of God. Love is constructive. It is free of fear.

Love overcomes obstacles and turns problems into opportunities for personal growth. Love, above all, is a desire to do good to others and to yourself. By its fruit, you shall know its value. The fruit of love is the help you give others.

Ask only what you can do to help others and the true nature of love will be obvious. Love is the ultimate spiritual lesson and gift. Give yourself the gift of understanding love.

Day 48

Practise 21 repetitions of each of the 5 limbering exercises plus 21 sit-ups.

Exercise

Choose your exercise mode and enjoy it.

Relaxation and Body Balancing

Read twice and then do.

For the first 3 minutes, relax and balance your body.

For the next 2 minutes repeat the power word for today: *reason.*

On a scale of 0 to 10, how well developed are your powers of reasoning?

Reflect on your answer and use creative imagery to evaluate your potential for further development of your ability to *reason*, reasonably.

Feel Good to Yourself
SYSTEMATIC PROBLEM SOLVING

Systematic problem solving will make you feel good quickly.

To do systematic problem solving, concentrate on one question at a time. Define the problem clearly in writing, maintaining an open mind and a sense of wonder. Use logic and positive language. See the problem as an opportunity or positive challenge.

Ask yourself all possible *causes* and list them. Then, identifying all conceivable solutions, make a decision as to which solution is your first priority. Assign responsibility for implementing the solution and set a deadline for accomplishing it.

Systematic problem solving will make you feel good about your use of logic or reason and it works!

Day 49

Practise 21 repetitions of each of the 5 limbering exercises plus 21 sit-ups.

Exercise

Choose your exercise mode and enjoy it.

Relaxation and Body Balancing

Read twice and then do.

For the first 3 minutes, relax and balance your body.

For the next 2 minutes repeat the power word for today: *wisdom*.

On a scale of 0 to 10, how wise are you?

Reflect on your answer and use creative imagery to evaluate your potential for further development of your wisdom, wisely.

Feel Good to Yourself
REFLECTION

Feeling good to yourself means taking time for reflection. The amount of time is not as critical as the quality of time spent in introspection.

Each day it is wise to reflect upon the events of that day. Be aware of unresolved emotional conflicts and decide how you can resolve them – before you go to bed. Never go to bed with a grudge.

Be aware also of the accomplishments of that day. Feel good about your virtues and the tasks well done, about development of greater patience, courage, fortitude and then set new goals for the next day, week or month.

Calm, peaceful introspection is a lovely way to feel good each day.

Day 50

Practise 21 repetitions of each of the 5 limbering exercises plus 21 sit-ups.

Exercise

Choose your exercise mode and enjoy it.

Relaxation and Body Balancing

Read twice and then do.

For the first 3 minutes, relax and balance your body.

For the next 2 minutes repeat the power word for today: *will.*

On a scale of 0 to 10, how strong is your will?

Reflect on your answer and use creative imagery to evaluate your potential for further development of your will.

Feel Good to Yourself
POWER

Feel good to yourself by reflecting upon your personal use of power. What does power mean to you – money, authority, prestige, or a sense of personal control? Does it include self-esteem? Does it include your right to choose your attitudes?

Do you stop at least once a month to assess your progress in reaching goals? Do you set your goals regularly and reassess their realism?

Do you respect your ability to think, to plan, to work towards these goals?

Do you bless yourself each day for all the wise choices you make? And for *learning* whenever you miss the mark?

In what other ways do you use the power of your will to feel good?

Day 51

Practise 21 repetitions of each of the 5 limbering exercises plus 21 sit-ups.

Today you may enjoy resting from your aerobic exercise routines.

Relaxation and Body Balancing

Read twice and then do.

For the first 3 minutes, relax and balance your body.

For the next 2 minutes repeat the power word for today: *faith*.

On a scale of 0 to 10, how strong is your faith?

Reflect on your answer and use creative imagery to evaluate your potential for further development of your faith.

Feel Good to Yourself
FAITH

Faith is a feel good blessing. Faith means that no matter what happens, you believe that the purpose of life is good. Faith is the belief that something good will arise from every crisis or major stress. Faith is the yeast for the bread of life. It allows you to rise from the ashes. Faith means finding *meaning* in life.

As Viktor Frankl said in *Man's Search for Meaning*, a sense of meaning or purpose is more important than starvation or typhus. And there must be meaning in life even if you don't know what it is, for anything else is insane. Faith is the only attitude which makes sense, and it feels good.

Day 52

Practise 21 repetitions of each of the 5 limbering exercises plus 21 sit-ups.

Exercise

Choose your exercise mode and enjoy it.

Relaxation and Body Balancing

Read twice and then do.

For the first 3 minutes, relax and balance your body.

For the next 2 minutes repeat the power word for today: *hope*.

On a scale of 0 to 10, how hopeful are you?

Reflect on your answer and use creative imagery to evaluate your potential for further development of your hope.

Feel Good to Yourself
HOPE

Hope is an essential feel good attitude. No matter how stressful the past has been, you can always hope the future will be better. Hope is the strength of the soul and spirit. It is the foundation for rising above distress.

Hope is an example of true love for yourself and others – a desire to *wish* good and do good. Just as the day follows night, opportunity for improvement most often comes with the challenges of life. When life presents you with lemons, hope allows you to make lemonade. Are you willing to reaffirm your hope each day – for success, for peace, for prosperity, for love?

Feel good by developing your hope.

Day 53

Practice 21 repetitions of each of the 5 limbering exercises plus 21 sit-ups.

Exercise

Choose your exercise mode and enjoy it.

Relaxation and Body Balancing

Read twice and then do.

For the first 3 minutes, relax and balance your body.

For the next 2 minutes repeat the power word for today: *charity*.

On a scale of 0 to 10, how charitable are you?

Reflect on your answer and use creative imagery to evaluate your potential for further development of your charitable instincts.

Feel Good to Yourself
HELP THE NEEDY

Feel good to yourself by helping those in need. No matter how serious life may seem to you, you can always find someone in greater need.

Rise out of the valley of self-indulgence to see the vast plains and mountains of human need. Focus your creativity upon solutions to the needs of others and find a greater wealth than imagined.

Great saints have usually risen to their highest potential through service to others. Learn the power of inner peace achieved when you assist others to smile, by comforting those in sorrow, by befriending the lonely. Much of the solution to human need is free for the giving – support, nurturing, encouragement, empathy, fulfilling your desire to do good.

FGTY by doing good to others.

Day 54

Practise 21 repetitions of each of the 5 limbering exercises plus 21 sit-ups.

Exercise

Choose your exercise mode and enjoy it.

Relaxation and Body Balancing

Read twice and then do.

For the first 3 minutes, relax and balance your body.

For the next 2 minutes repeat the power word for today: *courage.*

On a scale of 0 to 10, how courageous are you?

Reflect on your answer and use creative imagery to evaluate your potential for further development of your courage.

Feel Good to Yourself
THE COURAGE TO CHANGE

Feel good to yourself by exercising your courage to change.

True courage to change makes all other virtues possible. It provides the spiritual catalyst to produce change.

Recognize that change is essential to life. A real willingness to change implies a belief in yourself.

So when you find yourself in an unsatisfactory position, celebrate your strengths and use the opportunity to exercise the courage of change. Courage comes from excited enthusiasm about yourself, about the opportunity to make a difference. Overcome helplessness and fear of change by adopting a healthy courage to change those aspects of life which should be changed, and feel good about your courage.

Day 55

Practise 21 repetitions of each of the 5 limbering exercises plus 21 sit-ups.

Exercise

Choose your exercise mode and enjoy it.

Relaxation and Body Balancing

Read twice and then do.

For the first 3 minutes, relax and balance your body.

For the next 2 minutes repeat the power word for today: *joy*.

On a scale of 0 to 10, how joyous are you?

Reflect on your answer and use creative imagery to evaluate your potential for making yourself more joyous.

Feel Good to Yourself
JOY

Are you open to feeling joy about everything that happens to you? If you want to feel good, expect joy, experience joy, and express joy.

Practise for one day accepting everything that happens as a tiding of joy. Accept the happy message that God so loved the world that he gave his only begotten son, that they who believeth in Him, should not perish but have everlasting life. That is a great tiding of joy. Since

90 per cent of people believe in life after death and the survival of the soul, be aware that one of your major goals in life is to expect, feel and express joy. It feels good.

Day 56

Practise 21 repetitions of each of the 5 limbering exercises plus 21 sit-ups.

Exercise

Choose your exercise mode and enjoy it.

Relaxation and Body Balancing

Read twice and then do.

For the first 3 minutes, relax and balance your body.

For the next 2 minutes repeat the power word for today: *motivation.*

On a scale of 0 to 10, how motivated are you?

Reflect on your answer and use creative imagery to evaluate your potential for further development of your motivation.

Feel Good to Yourself
MOTIVATION

Motivation is an essential feel good attitude. Being motivated means putting enthusiasm and effort into whatever you do. Motivation means to strive to do a good job, to create success in any or all aspects of life, just for the pleasure of it. Motivation means taking responsibility for your welfare and for your thoughts and actions. Motivation means having a motive that is helpful to you while avoiding harm to others. It's having a zest for life, for work, for service, for love – having a desire to help others while feeling good to yourself. Reinforce your motivation daily with positive thoughts and actions.

Day 57

Practise 21 repetitions of each of the 5 limbering exercises plus 21 sit-ups.

Exercise

Choose your exercise mode and enjoy it.

Relaxation and Body Balancing

Read twice and then do.

For the first 3 minutes, relax and balance your body.

For the next 2 minutes repeat the power word for today: *confidence*.

On a scale of 0 to 10, how confident are you?

Reflect on your answer and use creative imagery to evaluate your potential for making yourself more confident.

Feel Good to Yourself
POSITIVE SELF-TALK

Recently I was talking with a psychologist who was facing the final exams for her doctorate.

'Can you imagine little me getting into this situation? What do I think I'm doing? I dread facing all those examiners who know so much more than I do and can ask me anything they please,' she said.

Oral exams are scary and I could appreciate her self-doubts, yet to do her best I knew she had to start thinking in a more positive direction. So I asked her to tell me about the subject of her dissertation, and she did. She became eloquent, confident, and interesting. After a few minutes, I interrupted her.

'I have learned so much just in these few minutes. How many of your examiners are going to know anything about this research?'

She smiled broadly and her body seemed taller and stronger. 'Really none,' she replied. 'You know, I feel really well prepared. It's going to work out.'

The lesson here is that frequently we can literally talk ourselves into success – and out of success even when we are ready and able. Do you talk to yourself to fail or to win?

Think about it and feel good by choosing to win.

Day 58

Practise 21 repetitions of each of the 5 limbering exercises plus 21 sit-ups.

This is a day to enjoy resting.

Relaxation and Body Balancing

Read twice and then do.

For the first 3 minutes, relax and balance your body.

For the next 2 minutes repeat the power word for today: *compassion*.

On a scale of 0 to 10, how compassionate are you?

Reflect on your answer and use creative imagery to evaluate your potential for making yourself more compassionate.

Feel Good to Yourself
MEANING

Feeling good requires a sense of purpose or meaning about life and the purpose of life. Although you may refine throughout life your thoughts in relation to this crucial issue, some general principles probably apply to most individuals. These include the concept of knowing there must be a purpose, for nothing else makes sense.

Beyond this basic wisdom, other attitudes which assist in feeling good include:

* Forgiveness towards those who offend you

* Tolerance for those with different beliefs

- Serenity despite the confusion of the world
- Compassion for all human beings
- Charity towards those less fortunate
- Hope that the future will be better
- Faith that the purpose in life is good
- Motivation to do your best
- Confidence that you can succeed
- Wisdom to make the best decision
- Reason in making decisions
- Love for yourself and others.

Day 59

Practise 21 repetitions of each of the 5 limbering exercises plus 21 sit-ups.

Exercise

Choose your exercise mode and enjoy it.

Relaxation and Body Balancing

Read twice and then do.

For the first 3 minutes, relax and balance your body.

For the next 2 minutes repeat the power word for today: *serenity*.

On a scale of 0 to 10, how serene are you?

Reflect on your answer and use creative imagery to evaluate your potential for making yourself more serene.

Feel Good to Yourself
AEQUINAMITAS

Feel good to yourself by developing aequinamitas. Sir William Osler, the father of American medicine, wrote his most inspirational essay on the topic of aequinamitas – the quality of being imperturbable.

Aequinamitas means coolness and presence of mind under all circumstances, calmness amid storm, clearness, judgment in moments of grave peril, immobility, impassiveness. It has the nature of a divine gift, a blessing – to all who come in contact with it.

Education, practice and experience are the major factors which allow you to become imperturbable. Use courage, calmness and serenity as the fundamental strengths of your feel good character.

Day 60

Practise 21 repetitions of each of the 5 limbering exercises plus 21 sit-ups.

Exercise

Choose your exercise mode and enjoy it.

Relaxation and Body Balancing

Read twice and then do.

For the first 3 minutes, relax and balance your body.

For the next 2 minutes repeat the power word for today: *tolerance*.

On a scale of 0 to 10, how tolerant are you?

Reflect on your answer and use creative imagery to evaluate your potential for making yourself more tolerant.

Feel Good to Yourself
VIRTUES

Feel good to yourself by developing those virtues you admire. Virtues build personality and enrich character.

Forgiveness, tolerance, patience, serenity, and goodwill are a few of the more common virtues. Make a list of all the traits, types of behaviour, and attitudes you consider virtuous. Then grade yourself on each of these. This gives you an opportunity to decide which ones are most needed in your own character.

Every day you have an opportunity to develop many different virtues. Whenever you encounter a problem, look upon it as an opportunity to exercise one or more virtuous qualities and feel good about your accomplishment.

Day 61

Practise 21 repetitions of each of the 5 limbering exercises plus 21 sit-ups.

Exercise

Choose your exercise mode and enjoy it.

Relaxation and Body Balancing

Read twice and then do.

For the first 3 minutes, relax and balance your body.

For the next 2 minutes repeat the power word for today: *patience*.

On a scale of 0 to 10, how patient are you?

Are you willing to be more patient with yourself and with others?

Reflect on your answer and use creative imagery to evaluate your potential for making yourself a more patient person.

Feel Good to Yourself
PATIENCE

Patience is a virtue that can help you feel good instead of feeling irritated.

Patience is the ability to endure pain, trouble, difficulty, and hardship without anger or irritation. Patience is also feeling calm and serene when the world around you seems chaotic. It is the ability to persevere and to put up with situations that are trying.

Patience is also a willingness to wait peacefully for the right time to complete a task or find an answer.

Patience is having the wisdom to know when to push hard and when to relax and detach.

Feel good by developing greater patience.

Day 62

Practise 21 repetitions of each of the 5 limbering exercises plus 21 sit-ups.

Exercise

Choose your exercise mode and enjoy it.

Relaxation and Body Balancing

Read twice and then do.

For the first 3 minutes, relax and balance your body.

For the next 2 minutes repeat the power word for today: *calm*.

On a scale of 0 to 10, how calm are you?

Reflect on your answer and use creative imagery to evaluate your potential for developing further a state of calm within yourself.

Feel Good to Yourself
TRANQUILLITY

Feel good by developing tranquillity. Tranquillity is the ability to be unperturbed by the storms of life; to be free of agitation.

Although it is essential that we become wise enough to recognize the differences between safe and unsafe, happy and unhappy, to discern harm from hurt, and desires from needs, agitation is not the solution to any problem. Tranquillity allows our intelligence to distinguish best from worst choices, to intuit and create solutions from turmoil.

Practise tranquillity any time life gives you the opportunity to detach from a seemingly chaotic situation. And each time you succeed in remaining tranquil, you'll feel good.

Day 63

Practise 21 repetitions of each of the 5 limbering exercises plus 21 sit-ups.

Exercise

Choose your exercise mode and enjoy it.

Relaxation and Body Balancing

Read twice and then do.

For the first 3 minutes, relax and balance your body.

For the next 2 minutes repeat the power word for today: *peace*.

On a scale of 0 to 10, how at peace are you?

Are you willing to be at peace just to feel good?

Reflect on your answer and use creative imagery to evaluate your potential for being at peace.

Feel Good to Yourself
PEACE

Feel good by creating a source of peace within. No other goal can accomplish so much for so many.

Peace is an attitude of freedom from noise, chaos, worry, fear, trouble.

Having a peaceful attitude does not mean denying problems; it simply means practising non-attachment to personal desires. It means avoiding desires to feel all right by substituting sex, power, or money for inner calm and wisdom.

Peace on earth requires goodwill toward others. Peace begins with forgiveness and tolerance, with patience, and with justified pride in detaching from fear. Just as the only fear we need to avoid is fear itself, the only peace we need begins inside each of us.

Feel good by being at peace.

Day 64

Practise 21 repetitions of each of the 5 limbering exercises plus 21 sit-ups.

Exercise

Choose your exercise mode and enjoy it.

Relaxation and Body Balancing

Read twice and then do.

For the first 3 minutes, relax and balance your body.

For the next 2 minutes repeat the power word for today: *bless*.

Before you begin, make a list of all those who have helped you in life.

See yourself sitting in front of them, one by one. Look into their eyes and say, 'Thank you. Bless you for all you have done for me.'

Feel yourself mean it.

Feel Good to Yourself
SPECIAL PEOPLE

Feel good to yourself by acknowledging the special people in your life. Tell them each day how much you like them and appreciate them. Show them that you care by your words and actions.

Be aware of the qualities you most like in your special friends or family. Do you share those qualities? Do you nurture these special relationships?

Do you share your innermost feelings with these special people? Do they understand you well?

Are you completely accepting and forgiving when this close group disagrees with you or acts in some way that you disapprove of?

If you really love these special people, do you act upon your desire to do good to them? Can you think of additional ways in which you might help them?

Feel good to yourself by acknowledging and nurturing the special people in your life.

Day 65

Practise 21 repetitions of each of the 5 limbering exercises plus 21 sit-ups.

Today you may enjoy resting from your aerobic exercise routine.

Relaxation and Body Balancing

Read twice and then do.

For the first 3 minutes, relax and balance your body.

For the next 2 minutes repeat the power word for today: *energy*.

What ideas, concepts, or 'causes' are worth great effort and energy? Make a list of those worth *your* energy.

Then after you are relaxed and balanced, grade these causes on a scale of 0 to 10. Which are you *willing* to solve?

Feel Good to Yourself
NEW OPPORTUNITIES

Feel good to yourself by creating new opportunities. There are virtually unlimited opportunities to create new jobs, new products, or new services.

When you observe a problem of any kind, examine what is missing, then you can seek a solution. And as you work towards a solution, each day will bring new opportunities to expand your horizons.

The world presents a feast of opportunities and new ways to do good to yourself and to others. So feel good to yourself by taking advantage of the many opportunities provided.

Day 66

Practise 21 repetitions of each of the 5 limbering exercises plus 21 sit-ups.

Exercise

Choose your exercise mode and enjoy it.

Relaxation and Body Balancing

Read twice and then do.

For the first 3 minutes, relax and balance your body.

For the next 2 minutes repeat the power word for today: *separate*.

Be aware of your connections to your family and its ancient roots. How do they hinder you? How do they help you? What strings of attachment are there? Are you willing to separate yourself? If so, see yourself cutting those strings.

Feel Good to Yourself
DEVELOPING YOUR FAMILY TREE

Feel good to yourself by building upon the best of your ethnic roots. Each of us represents the current stage of evolution of our social and ethnic ancestry. And every culture throughout history has included both mature and immature behaviour.

What do you know about your family tree? If you feel any shame about any limb of your tree, can you develop that virtue representing the more mature version of that trait? And for those aspects of your ancestry which evoke pride, are you continuing to cultivate and express them?

No matter what the twigs and flowers of your family tree, you can work to be the best, most responsible, wisest person you know.

Feel good to yourself by using your family history for personal growth.

Day 67

Practise 21 repetitions of each of the 5 limbering exercises plus 21 sit-ups.

Exercise

Choose your exercise mode and enjoy it.

Relaxation and Body Balancing

Read twice and then do.

For the first 3 minutes, relax and balance your body.

For the next 2 minutes repeat the power word for today: *detach*.

Be aware of your connections to your country or nation and its ancient roots. How do they hinder you? How do they help you? What strings of attachment are there? Are you willing to separate yourself? If so, see yourself cutting those strings.

Feel Good to Yourself
SOCIAL SURROUNDINGS

Feel good to yourself by comparing the influences of your social surroundings upon you.

Be aware of the influences upon your personality of your great-grandparents, your grandparents, your parents, and your siblings. How does the ancient culture of your ancestors affect you today? Suppose just one person of your family tree had been different – how would that change have influenced you? How does the culture of your town, school, county, or state influence your perception of reality? How different are you because of being born in your home country compared with someone born in some other country or on some other continent?

How different are you because you were born in the twentieth century instead of the nineteenth or even earlier?

Feel good to yourself by being aware of the many factors which make you.

Day 68

Practise 21 repetitions of each of the 5 limbering exercises plus 21 sit-ups.

Exercise

Choose your exercise mode and enjoy it.

Relaxation and Body Balancing

Read twice and then do.

For the first 3 minutes, relax and balance your body.

For the next 2 minutes repeat the power word for today: *detach.*

Be aware of your connections to your religion and its ancient roots. How do they hinder you? How do they help you? What strings of attachment are there? Are you willing to separate yourself? If so, see yourself cutting those strings.

Feel Good to Yourself
RELIGIOUS BELIEFS

Feel good to yourself by evaluating your religious beliefs. Religion is one social expression of spiritual values. And although all great religions share certain beliefs, especially about the golden rule (see page 8), most also include dogma handed down in writing and interpreted by clergy or by you.

Is your interpretation similar to that of your clergy? Of your religion? Are the rituals meaningful to you? Do they produce guilt or ecstasy? Does your religion allow for freedom of thought and actions compatible with *your* beliefs? Above all, does your religion demonstrate the fruits of forgiveness, of tolerance, of truly doing good to others?

Feel good to yourself by expressing your spiritual values appropriately.

Day 69

Practise 21 repetitions of each of the 5 limbering exercises plus 21 sit-ups.

Exercise

Choose your exercise mode and enjoy it.

Relaxation and Body Balancing

Read twice and then do.

For the first 3 minutes, relax and balance your body.

For the next 2 minutes repeat the power word for today: *secure*.

How secure are you in your sexuality? Do you like being your sex?

Be aware of the advantages.

Be aware of the disadvantages.

Feel Good to Yourself
SEXUALITY

Feel good to yourself by exploring your sexuality. What does *being* your sex mean to you?

What are the special responsibilities and opportunities offered by being your sex. What are the problems or shortcomings of being your sex? How does your sexuality relate to your sense of power? Of strength? Of career? Of roles is life? What does your sexuality deprive you of? Or assist you in?

Is being your sex a feel good aspect of your life? What can you do to improve your feelings about your sexuality?

Day 70

Practise 21 repetitions of each of the 5 limbering exercises plus 21 sit-ups.

Exercise

Choose your exercise mode and enjoy it.

Relaxation and Body Balancing

Read twice and then do.

For the first 3 minutes, relax and balance your body.

For the next 2 minutes repeat the power word for today: *secure*.

How secure are you in your sexuality? Can you imagine having sex with your best male friend?

Explore the images and feelings.

Feel Good to Yourself
YOUR SEXUAL REALITY

Feel good to yourself by exploring your sexual reality.

Recall the first time you were ever sexually aroused. What were the circumstances? Was anyone else involved or were you alone? Was the entire experience pleasurable?

What types of situations turn you on sexually? Are you sexually aroused by:

  Yourself
  Your best friend of the opposite sex

Your best friend of your own sex
Only by the opposite sex
Only by your own sex
Equally by both sexes.

Is sex a fun experience for you? Do you enjoy pleasing yourself sexually? Is sexual activity a spiritual experience?

FGTY by enhancing your sexual satisfaction.

Day 71

Practise 21 repetitions of each of the 5 limbering exercises plus 21 sit-ups.

Exercise

Choose your exercise mode and enjoy it.

Relaxation and Body Balancing

Read twice and then do.

For the first 3 minutes, relax and balance your body.

For the next 2 minutes repeat the power word for today: *secure*.

How secure are you in your sexuality? Can you imagine having sex with your best female friend?

Explore the images and feelings.

Feel Good to Yourself
SEXUALITY

Feel good to yourself by exploring your sexuality.

What are your sexual dreams? Fantasies? Do you spend time creating fun fantasies – or guilty ones?

Are your fantasies compatible with your ethics, your commitments?

Are you sexually aroused by reading or seeing pornography? Are you sexually aroused by *yourself?*

If you can turn yourself on, does that make you bisexual? Freud believed everyone has a bisexual capability. Can you be turned on by *anyone* of your own sex?

Suppose you were isolated for months or years only with someone of your own sex. Would you then prefer *mutual* to self sex?

Is it ever acceptable to 'have' sex with anyone other than your spouse?

Feel good to yourself by contemplating the breadth and depth of your sexual feelings.

Day 72

Practise 21 repetitions of each of the 5 limbering exercises plus 21 sit-ups.

Today choose to enjoy resting.

Relaxation and Body Balancing

Read twice and then do.

For the first 3 minutes, relax and balance your body.

For the next 2 minutes repeat the power word for today: *sex.*

If you can enjoy masturbation, you can be turned on by someone of your own sex! In situations where sexes are isolated, same sex activity is very common. Reflect on your ability to be aroused by either sex.

Feel Good to Yourself
SEXUALITY

Feel good to yourself by understanding your sexuality.

Wilhelm Reich has said that you can't really have enjoyable sex with anyone else until you can satisfy yourself!

Do you really know how to satisfy yourself? What turns you on? When? What turns you off? Why? Are you sexually aroused by words, thoughts, memories, images, feelings? What parts of your body *feel* sexually? Can you be aroused by touching yourself – on your thighs, abdomen, breasts, lips? Can you be aroused by looking at yourself?

Take time to feel, see, hear, taste, smell and *know* yourself sexually. And don't forget to *please* yourself! That's real feel good.

Day 73

Practise 21 repetitions of each of the 5 limbering exercises plus 21 sit-ups.

Exercise

Choose your exercise mode and enjoy it.

Relaxation and Body Balancing

Read twice and then do.

For the first 3 minutes, relax and balance your body.

For the next 2 minutes repeat the power word for today: *secure*.

How secure are you financially? What are your fears related to money? How much power/energy do you devote to worrying about money?

Feel Good to Yourself
ANXIETY

Feel good to yourself by controlling your anxiety. There are many ways to avoid and overcome anxiety.

First and foremost, is the worry really worth your energy? Most people appear to become anxious about *possibilities*, not *probabilities*.

Ask yourself: can I settle the problem by worrying? If not, can I divorce it with joy? And finally, am I willing to accept and forgive? Go for sainthood and be at peace.

Beyond such rational thinking, exercise vigorously. A 30 minute jog is more relaxing than a tranquillizer and much safer!

And finally, just practise deep relaxation – focus your attention on *any* thought that is pleasant and you'll feel good and be free of anxiety.

Day 74

Practise 21 repetitions of each of the 5 limbering exercises plus 21 sit-ups.

Exercise

Choose your exercise mode and enjoy it.

Relaxation and Body Balancing

Read twice and then do.

For the first 3 minutes, relax and balance your body.

For the next 2 minutes repeat the power word for today: *responsibility*.

How responsible are you? do you take full responsibility for your thoughts and actions?

Feel Good to Yourself
RESPONSIBILITY

Feel good to yourself by exercising your sense of responsibility. When you accept a duty or task, you have become responsible for satisfactory completion. Each of us has many responsibilities in life, all revolving around one basic principle: to perform our activities without harming anyone else.

The first lesson is avoiding harm; the second is being of service to others.

We also have responsibilities to ourselves – to treat our bodies as a holy temple; to use our minds intelligently and wisely; to develop those aspects of personality and character we consider virtues; to treat ourselves as well as we treat everyone else.

Accepting these responsibilities is a wise way to feel good.

Day 75

Practise 21 repetitions of each of the 5 limbering exercises plus 21 sit-ups.

Exercise

Choose your exercise mode and enjoy it.

Relaxation and Body Balancing

Read twice and then do.

For the first 3 minutes, relax and balance your body.

For the next 2 minutes repeat the power word for today: *responsibility*.

Do you have any resentments towards others who have failed to accept responsibility? Do you need to confront them? Are you willing to forgive them?

Feel Good to Yourself
RESPONSIBILITY

Feel good to yourself by evaluating your sense of responsibility.

Be aware of where your personal responsibility begins and ends. In general, your major responsibility is to avoid harming others with your actions or words. Beyond that basic responsibility, the choice is yours. You have a right to choose or refuse most other responsibilities.

When you choose a job, you accept specific duties and responsibilities. Be careful you don't bite off more than you can chew. When you choose to have children or acquire a pet, you take on new responsibilities. When you marry, give or accept friendship, you choose different responsibilities.

Everyone has responsibilities, but you are responsible only for your own. If someone else fails in their responsibility and you choose to do it for them, feel good and be happy with your choice. On a scale of 0 to 10, how happy are you?

Day 76

Practise 21 repetitions of each of the 5 limbering exercises plus 21 sit-ups.

Exercise

Choose your exercise mode and enjoy it.

Relaxation and Body Balancing

Read twice and then do.

For the first 3 minutes, relax and balance your body.

For the next 2 minutes repeat the power word for today: *forgive*.

Do you have any guilt over any past action or thoughts? Is there anything you should do to make amends? Are you ready to forgive yourself?

Feel Good to Yourself
LOVE YOUR NEIGHBOUR

Feel good to yourself by loving your neighbour as yourself.

No one is perfect. When you notice flaws in your neighbour, do not criticize, but say, 'Here, let me help you'. Rejoice at the successes of your neighbour and bless them for the good they do. Remember that loving someone means only desiring to do good to them.

Are you forgiving when your neighbour says or does something annoying? Are you tolerant of your neighbour's difference from you? Can you rejoice in the beauty of diversity? Are you at peace with your neighbour?

And remember to be forgiving, tolerant, and at peace with yourself.

Do good to yourself and your neighbour and you will have fulfilled the most essential spiritual goal. Feel good by desiring good for your neighbour and yourself.

Day 77

Practise 21 repetitions of each of the 5 limbering exercises plus 21 sit-ups.

Exercise

Choose your exercise mode and enjoy it.

Relaxation and Body Balancing

Read twice and then do.

For the first 3 minutes, relax and balance your body.

For the next 2 minutes repeat the power word for today: *love*.

Can you look in the mirror and say, 'I love you', and mean it? Say, 'I'm all right because God does not make rubbish.'

Sense, see, feel, know that you accept and love yourself.

Feel Good to Yourself
TREAT YOURSELF WELL

Charity begins at home! Feel good by choosing to treat yourself well so that you can do a better job of helping others.

Can you imagine going through an entire day saying to yourself, 'I love you'? And meaning it?

Start your day by looking in a mirror and affirming your desire first and foremost to do good to yourself! Not to treat yourself as *better* than anyone else – just to treat yourself *as well* as you treat others.

And if you don't like yourself, change your thoughts and actions to those you do like. Say to yourself, 'I'm all right because God does not create rubbish.'

Exercise your will by developing attitudes and attributes that you respect and admire. Then you'll be most effective in doing good to others as well as to yourself.

Day 78

Practise 21 repetitions of each of the 5 limbering exercises plus 21 sit-ups.

Exercise

Choose your exercise mode and enjoy it.

Relaxation and Body Balancing

Read twice and then do.

For the first 3 minutes, relax and balance your body.

For the next 2 minutes repeat the power word for today: *wisdom*.

Once you are relaxed and balanced, imagine you are standing on the top of a beautiful mountain. In front of you is a pleasant fire; beside you is the wisest person in the world. Ask your wise friend the most important question you have. Listen carefully and understand the answer.

Feel Good to Yourself
LISTENING TO THE INNER STILLNESS

Feel good to yourself by learning to hear the quiet stillness of your inner self, of the *real* you.

First you need to practise detachment from concerns and worries outside you. And to quieten the clatter of your mind. This may require many days of practising the art of focusing attention on one thought at a time.

Gradually as you improve your quality of focusing, you can ask yourself a simple question and wait patiently for an answer. Often the answer will not come at that time, but will pop into your mind later when you least 'expect' it.

The more you practise, the more often you will receive effective answers. When the truth comes, you will know it intuitively and as certainly as any fact of the universe.

Feel good to yourself by listening in peace and harmony.

Day 79

Practise 21 repetitions of each of the 5 limbering exercises plus 21 sit-ups.

This is a day to enjoy resting.

Relaxation and Body Balancing

Read twice and then do.

For the first 3 minutes, relax and balance your body.

For the next 2 minutes repeat the power word for today: *forgive*.

Make a list of all the people who have harmed or hurt you. One by one, see yourself sitting in front of them. Look into their eyes and say – and mean it – 'I forgive you'.

Feel yourself forgive them.

Feel Good to Yourself
GO WITH THE FLOW

Feel good to yourself by learning to 'go with the flow'.

We all experience stress when we feel threatened. Threats, real or perceived, trigger the 'fight or flight' response. But most threats do not really threaten our lives. Indeed, they rarely threaten our health, except through anxiety, anger, or depression.

'Threats' may be as minor as a snide comment. Other people's words do not harm me; my thoughts do. 'Sticks and stones may break my bones' and indeed *should* trigger fight or flight. But words are rarely actions; they need not set off an alarm reaction.

While you don't have to put up with physical or verbal abuse, what are your choices when someone attacks you or maligns you verbally?

You can talk back – in a note, an argument, or a lawsuit. That is verbal fighting. You can separate yourself – 'divorce' them. That is flight. Or you can *consider the source* – separate, detach, accept, forgive, smile. Feel good by going with the flow.

Day 80

Practise 21 repetitions of each of the 5 limbering exercises plus 21 sit-ups.

Exercise

Choose your exercise mode and enjoy it.

Relaxation and Body Balancing

Read twice and then do.

For the first 3 minutes, relax and balance your body.

For the next 2 minutes repeat the power word for today: *love*.

Create a sense of complete desire to do good to yourself and others. Sense, see, feel, hear, taste, smell unconditional love for every living being.

Feel Good to Yourself
PEOPLE WATCHING

Feel good to yourself by spending a few hours just observing people – in the high street or at a beach, at a park or in school.

Just sit or stand and observe. Watch carefully their clothes, their size, their posture, their sex. Note their jewellery, the colours of their clothes, of their skin. The colours of their hair, of their eyes. Listen to the *meaning* of their sounds.

Notice especially their facial expressions and the meaning of their 'body language'. Can you imagine how their parents look, what they do for a living, how angry or happy they are? Can you sense their fears and their ability to love? Can you feel compassion for each person you see? Can you feel unconditional love? A desire to do good to them?

FGTY by sensing your relation to other people.

Day 81

Practise 21 repetitions of each of the 5 limbering exercises plus 21 sit-ups.

Exercise

Choose your exercise mode and enjoy it.

Relaxation and Body Balancing

Read twice and then do.

For the first 3 minutes, relax and balance your body.

For the next 2 minutes repeat the power word for today: *express*.

Are you ready to communicate your needs and desires: your will to live; your will to survive; your will to nurture and be nurtured? Reflect on what it takes to express yourself fully.

Feel Good to Yourself
SELF-IMAGE

Feel good to yourself by exploring your image of yourself. If you were describing yourself to a stranger, what 10 adjectives would you use to describe your most prominent attitudes? If your closest friends were describing you, what 10 adjectives would they use?

If you were describing your physical appearance, what adjectives would you use? How do you feel about your clothes? Your weight? Your posture?

How helpful are you? How cooperative? Are you willing and able to compromise when your opinion differs from that of friends, co-workers, family? Do you care enough about those around you to listen?

What is your major role in life? Hero/ine, warrior, parent, politician, peacemaker, star, or supporter?

Do you feel good about the image you have created?

Day 82

Practise 21 repetitions of each of the 5 limbering exercises plus 21 sit-ups.

Exercise

Choose your exercise mode and enjoy it.

Relaxation and Body Balancing

Read twice and then do.

For the first 3 minutes, relax and balance your body.

For the next 2 minutes repeat the power word for today: *knowing*.

Concentrate on quietening the idle chatter of your mind and listen to the small quiet voice within.

Are you willing to accept your *intuition*, your intrinsic knowledge about the most important questions you have about life?

Feel Good to Yourself
YOUR INTUITIVE POWER

Feel good to yourself by using your intuition. When you get up in the morning, how do you *know* what to wear, what to eat for breakfast? How do you choose the right road to work or even the type of career you will pursue? What do your instincts tell you about food, people, friends, and family? Do you use intuition to help you in making your choices in life?

How accurate is your intuition? Is it based upon fear or detached wise knowing?

If you learn to focus your mind, to concentrate on one chosen thought or idea, to listen to the quiet still voice within, you can enhance your intuition. Some individuals have a natural intuitive ability that is greater than average, just as some musicians have natural ability. But all of us have intuition.

FGTY by honouring your intuitive power.

Day 83

Practise 21 repetitions of each of the 5 limbering exercises plus 21 sit-ups.

Exercise

Choose your exercise mode and enjoy it.

Relaxation and Body Balancing

Read twice and then do.

For the first 3 minutes, relax and balance your body.

For the next 2 minutes repeat the power word for today: *divine*.

Be aware of the divine nature of your inner being, your higher self, your soul. Sense, know, say, and mean 'I know at my innermost being I am magnificent, wise, and loving'.

Create an image of a giant sky-blue, five-pointed star beaming down upon you.

Feel Good to Yourself
YOU ARE YOUR SOUL

Feel good to yourself by recognizing that you are not your body. You are not your muscles, bones, organs, or blood. You are not even your mind, your ego, or your emotions. Recognize that you are the inner centre of consciousness of your soul.

When you accept the reality of being a unique, divine soul, you acknowledge your responsibility for using your inner wisdom. In this way you will choose thoughts, actions, and habits that use the power of your body, mind, and emotions to create total health and good for yourself and others.

Allow your inner higher being to transform your doubts and fears with the illumination of divine love. Focus your awareness on attunement with your true self and feel good every moment of every day.

Aung Slm Sun Kyc, the 1991 Nobel Peace Prize Laureate, said in the *Wall Street Journal Europe*: The quintessential revolution is that of spirit . . . the realization of this depends solely upon human responsibility. At the root of that responsibility lies the concept of perfection, the urge to achieve it, the intelligence to find a path toward it, and the will to follow that path if not to the end, at least the distance needed to rise above individual limitation.

Day 84

Practise 21 repetitions of each of the 5 limbering exercises plus 21 sit-ups.

Exercise

Choose your exercise mode and enjoy it.

Relaxation and Body Balancing

Read twice and then do.

For the first 3 minutes, relax and balance your body.

For the next 2 minutes repeat the power word for today: *power*.

Be aware of the divine nature of the universe and of your connectedness to God. Create an image of a giant white six-pointed star beaming a golden-orange light upon you.

Feel Good to Yourself
POWER

Feel good to yourself by enhancing your personal sense of power. Power is your inner reserve or strength to think straight, to exercise discernment, to feel all right about yourself.

Power is your willingness to work on yourself, to develop virtues, to persist in your goals.

Power is having the wisdom to make choices that work well for you.

Power is freedom from anger, guilt and worry. It is having confidence in yourself and motivation to persevere.

Power is knowing that you can succeed. It is the foundation for good self-esteem.

Feel good by exercising your inner power.

Day 85

Practise 21 repetitions of each of the 5 limbering exercises plus 21 sit-ups.

Exercise

Choose your exercise mode and enjoy it.

Relaxation and Body Balancing

Read twice and then do.

For the first 3 minutes, relax and balance your body.

For the next 2 minutes repeat the power word for today: *right*.

Is my conduct the result of a specific moral code? How do I define my moral beliefs?

Feel Good to Yourself
RIGHT AND WRONG

Feel good to yourself by exploring your concepts of 'right' and 'wrong'. *Who* decides what is right or wrong? Is it your parents, 'the law', or God? Who speaks for God? When we hear and read the remarkable differences in beliefs about God, who has the truth? Can the Arabs and the Israelis both be right? – or wrong? How about the Irish Protestants versus the Catholics?

Is it ever right to rob, steal, abuse, murder?

Are you willing to base your feelings – beliefs – about right and wrong, whenever possible, on that which harms no one?

Feel good to yourself by living the golden rule. Think and feel – is this action free of harm to myself and others?

Day 86

Practise 21 repetitions of each of the 5 limbering exercises plus 21 sit-ups.

Today you may enjoy resting.

Relaxation and Body Balancing

Read twice and then do.

For the first 3 minutes, relax and balance your body.

For the next 2 minutes repeat the power word for today: *spirit*.

Do I believe in prayer? Do I pray to ask for some gift for myself or others? Or do I pray in thanksgiving? Or do I pray in awe of the divine?

Feel Good to Yourself
PRAYER

Feel good to yourself with the power of prayer. Even though 'every thought is a prayer', you can improve your health by focusing each day on thoughts aimed at peace and love.

The greatest benefit of prayer may be the benefit of relaxation. Prayer is not a time of presenting a wish list, but rather is a time for savouring and appreciating blessings – and for sharing a hope of blessing with those in need.

Consider having a long period of prayer each morning when you awaken.

Be thankful and joyous for the opportunity to begin another day of service. Set your mood for the day as one of peace and love – a desire to do good to others.

And end your day the same way, being thankful for the opportunity of that day and preparing yourself for a feel good sleep by putting yourself at peace with every event of that day.

Day 87

Practice 21 repetitions of each of the 5 limbering exercises plus 21 sit-ups.

Exercise

Choose your favourite exercise mode and enjoy it.

Relaxation and Body Balancing

Read twice and then do.

For the first 3 minutes, relax and balance your body.

For the next 2 minutes repeat the power word for today: *meaning*.

What is my life's purpose? Do I have a spiritual purpose in life?

Feel Good to Yourself
PUT MEANING IN LIFE

Feel good to yourself by taking time to reflect upon the meaning of your life. Ultimately, for most persons, meaning implies a spiritual value. As Evelyn Underhill said, 'Living the spiritual life is the attitude you hold in your mind when you're down on your knees scrubbing the steps.'

Have you examined your sense of meaning lately? Are you aware of your attitude upon awakening, when you greet your family, when you eat your meals, when you drive or walk to work? Are you aware of your attitude all day at work? In the evening?

Do you pay attention to your attitude and sense of meaning – or escape with meaning*less* activity? Do you use television to avoid thinking and changing? Are you willing to be responsible for putting meaning into your life?

Day 88

Practise 21 repetitions of each of the 5 limbering exercises plus 21 sit-ups.

Exercise

Choose your favourite exercise mode and enjoy it.

Relaxation and Body Balancing

Read twice and then do.

For the first 3 minutes, relax and balance your body.

For the next 2 minutes repeat the power word for today: *soul.*

Do I believe in a soul – a higher self? Do I believe that the essence of my being, my soul, survives the death of my physical body?

Feel Good to Yourself
WHO ARE YOU

Feel good to yourself by reflecting on who you are. Tune in to the various parts of your body, systematically from toes to head.

- Are you your feet, your legs, or your sexual organs?

- Are you your abdomen, with its vast chemical factory?

- Are you your back, your chest, your lungs or heart?

- Are you your shoulders, arms, hands, or fingers?

- Are you your neck, or your face, eyes, nose, ears, mouth?

- Are you your brain, your skin or your hair?

Can you recognize that your body, wonderful though it is, is only the temple in which you live?

Repeat several times to yourself, 'I have a body which I love dearly and treat well. I live in my body and appreciate it.'

Feel good to yourself by saying and feeling, 'I am more than my body.'

Day 89

Practice 21 repetitions of each of the 5 limbering exercises plus 21 sit-ups.

Exercise

Choose your favourite exercise mode and enjoy it.

Relaxation and Body Balancing

Read twice and then do.

For the first 3 minutes, relax and balance your body.

For the next 2 minutes repeat the power word for today: *God.*

Do I believe in God? How do I see, feel, *know* God?

Do I believe that God is a luminous, perfect, omnipotent soul or some other unifying power?

Feel Good to Yourself
ACKNOWLEDGE THE DIVINE

Feel good to yourself by recognizing the divinity of all creation. Be aware that God created every atom of the universe. Thus every rock and mineral is sacred. Every plant, animal, and human being is a spark of the divine.

Seek the inner perfection in all you see, hear, taste, smell, and feel. Be aware that at some level there is a perfect manifestation awaiting discovery.

The universal power we call God is the source of all energy. Explore the hidden sacred message in each aspect of creation. Respect and revere the beauty and magnificence of the universe and of the earth, of all creation.

Focus your energy upon reflecting the divinity inherent within.

FGTY by acknowledging the sacred.

Day 90

Practise 21 repetitions of each of the 5 limbering exercises plus 21 sit-ups.

Exercise

Choose your favourite exercise mode and enjoy it.

Relaxation and Body Balancing

Read twice and then do.

For the first 3 minutes, relax and balance your body.

For the next 2 minutes repeat the power word for today: *service*.

Do I believe in service to others? How do I focus my energy to achieve service? How much of my total energy is spent on me? My family? My friends? Those less fortunate than I? Reflect on these thoughts from *My Dear Alexias*:

> . . . the luxury of self-centred grief, 'walking in the twilight', not only engenders mental and physical depression; but actually retards the progress and well-being of the loved one for whom you grieve. To help others . . . one must walk in the sunlight and pour its radiance into the twilight regions where grief, resentment and self-centred sorrows abide. This cannot be done if one descends oneself.

Feel Good to Yourself
CHARITABLE GIVING

Feel good to yourself with your charitable gifts. The best gift is yourself. The greatest gift need cost nothing except time and enthusiasm. Think about all the wonderful projects which contribute to the welfare of those less fortunate that you. Each of us will have special attractions to one or more causes. Giving money is always helpful, but providing your personal energy and creativity can be even more rewarding to you and the receiver.

Volunteer to help a charitable organization, to assist a neighbour in need, to befriend a child or adult. The attitude you hold is the spiritual gift. Choose an attitude of giving yourself to feel good.

Conclusion

It takes about three months to become habituated. Hopefully, by now, you are habituated to relaxing, balancing body tension, resolving conflicts, having insight into your self, and being at peace.

Obviously any of the previous exercises can be used again and again to reach ever deeper into yourself. Some individuals will move into ever more perfect meditation and attunement with the divine. Some will use their new power to further creativity and intuition.

Commit yourself to repeat the entire programme four times a year or create a plan *each day* for relaxation, motivation (power word), and contemplation or meditation.

And don't forget physical exercise!

Further Reading

Assagioli, Roberto, *Psychosynthesis*, The Viking Press, New York, NY, 1971.

Bailey, Alice A., *Esoteric Healing*, Vol. IV, Lucis Publishing Co., London, 1953.

Barlow, Wilfred, *The Alexander Technique*, Alfred A. Knopf, New York, NY, 1977.

Bates, W. H., *The Bates Method For Better Eyesight Without Glasses*, Pyramid Books, New York, NY.

Benson, Herbert, *The Relaxation Response*, William Morrow & Co., New York, NY, 1975.

Bonny, Helen L., and Louis M. Savary, *Music and Your Mind: Listening With A New Consciousness*, Harper & Row, New York, NY, 1973.

Boston Women's Health Book Collection, *Our Bodies, Ourselves*, Simon & Schuster, New York, NY, 2nd ed., 1984.

Cooper, Kenneth H., MD, *Aerobics*, Bantam Books, New York, NY, 1968.

Cooper, Kenneth H., MD, *The Aerobics Way*, Bantam Books, New York, NY, 1981.

Cooper, Kenneth H., MD, *The Aerobics Program for Total Well-Being*, M. Evans, New York, NY, 1902.

Cooper, Kenneth H., MD, *Running Without Fear: How to Reduce the Risk of Heart Attack and Sudden Death during Aerobic Exercise*, M. Evans, New York, NY, 1985.

Cooper, Kenneth H., MD, *Kid Fitness: A Complete Shape-Up Program from Birth Through High School*, Bantam, New York, NY, 1991.

Fox, Arnold, MD, *The Beverly Hills Medical Diet*, Chain-Pinkham Books, St Louis Park, MN, 1981.

Frankl, Viktor E., *Man's Search for Meaning*, Beacon Press, Boston, MA, 1959.

Gallwey, W. Timothy, *The Inner Game of Tennis*, Bantam Books, New York, NY, 1974.

Gaythorpe, Elizabeth (ed.), *My Dear Alexias: Letters from Wellesley Tudor Pole to Rosamond Lehmann*, Neville Spearman, Jersey, Channel Islands, 1979.

Harris, Thomas A., *I'm OK – You're OK: A Practical Guide to Transactional Analysis*, Harper & Row, New York, NY, 1967.

Hill, Napoleon, *Think and Grow Rich*, Ballantine Books, New York, NY, 1988 (Copyright 1960).

Holmes, T. H. and Rahe, R. H., 'The Social Readjustment Rating Scale', *Journal of Psychosomatic Research*, 11: 213–18, 1967.

Hudson, Thomson Jay, *The Law of Psychic Phenomena*, Samuel Weiser, Inc., New York, NY, 1968.

Jacobson, Edmund, *Progressive Relaxation*, The University of Chicago Press, Chicago, IL, Midway Reprint, 1974.

Knowles, John, 'The Responsibility of the Individual', *Daedalus*, Winter issue, 1977: 57–80.

McKeown, Thomas, *The Role of Medicine: Dream, Mirage or Nemesis*, Nuffield Provincial Hospitals Trust, England, 1976.

Osler, Sir William, *Aequanimitas*, McGraw-Hill Book Co., New York, NY, 2nd ed, 1932.

Pelletier, Kenneth R., *Mind As Healer, Mind As Slayer*, Delacorte Press, New York, NY, 1977.

Selye, Hans, *Stress Without Distress*, J. B. Lippincott Co., Philadelphia, PA, 1974.

Shealy, C. Norman, *Miracles Do Happen*, Element Books, Boston, MA, 1996.

Smith, Manuel, J., PhD, *When I Say No, I Feel Guilty*, Bantam Books, New York, NY, 1975. (Originally published by Dial Press 1975.)

Underhill, Evelyn, *The Spiritual Life*, Harper & Row, New York, NY, 1976.

Wilbanks, William Lee, 'The New Obscenity', *Vital Speeches of the Day*, 15 August 1988. 389 Highway 17 By-Pass, Mt. Pleasant, South Carolina 29464.

Woods, Margo, *Masturbation, Tantra and Self Love*, Omphaloskepsis Press, San Diego, CA, 1981.

Worrall, Ambrose Alexander, *Essay on Prayer*, Self-Health Systems, Fair Grove, Missouri. (Originally published Baltimore 1952.)

Zilbergeld, Bernie, *Male Sexuality*, Bantam Books, New York, NY, 1978.